T0115174

Prevention Does Work: A Guide to a Healthy Heart

A Cardiologist and a Cook Present the Facts and the Foods

PAUL GOLDFINGER, MD, FACC,
AND EILEEN GOLDFINGER

iUniverse, Inc.
Bloomington

Prevention Does Work: A Guide to a Healthy Heart
A Cardiologist and a Cook Present the Facts and the Foods

Copyright © 2011 Paul Goldfinger, MD, FACC, and Eileen Goldfinger

All rights reserved. No part of this book may be used or reproduced by any means, graphic, electronic, or mechanical, including photocopying, recording, taping or by any information storage retrieval system without the written permission of the publisher except in the case of brief quotations embodied in critical articles and reviews.

The information, ideas, and suggestions in this book are not intended as a substitute for professional medical advice. Before following any suggestions contained in this book, you should consult your personal physician. Neither the author nor the publisher shall be liable or responsible for any loss or damage allegedly arising as a consequence of your use or application of any information or suggestions in this book.

iUniverse books may be ordered through booksellers or by contacting:

iUniverse
1663 Liberty Drive
Bloomington, IN 47403
www.iuniverse.com
1-800-Authors (1-800-288-4677)

Because of the dynamic nature of the Internet, any Web addresses or links contained in this book may have changed since publication and may no longer be valid. The views expressed in this work are solely those of the author and do not necessarily reflect the views of the publisher, and the publisher hereby disclaims any responsibility for them.

Any people depicted in stock imagery provided by Thinkstock are models, and such images are being used for illustrative purposes only.

Certain stock imagery © Thinkstock.

ISBN: 978-1-4620-0061-6 (pbk)
ISBN: 978-1-4620-0062-3 (cloth)
ISBN: 978-1-4620-0063-0 (ebk)

Printed in the United States of America

iUniverse rev. date: 3/10/2011

Contents

Preface

Prevention does work. We are referring to the scientific progress made over the last sixty years in the prevention of cardiovascular disease, a condition which causes many deaths and much disability in this country.

Paul Goldfinger, MD, FACC, is a cardiologist who is board certified in both internal medicine and cardiology, He has been on the faculty of two medical schools and he has published scientific papers in the medical literature. Dr. Goldfinger has been interested in prevention for many years, especially the nutritional aspects. When it became clear that prevention methods were saving lives, he decided that physicians were not doing enough to educate their patients about prevention. He also became aware that people did not know how to prepare heart-healthy meals at home. He enlisted the help of his wife, Eileen Goldfinger, an experienced cook who learned the nutritional principles along with him, and they collaborated to design a unique patient education book that was both an information source for lay people and a heart-healthy cookbook.

"Prevention Does Work" has been popular with patients and healthcare providers. The "two books in one" concept is a unique and practical idea. This is the fourth and most complete version. It is hoped that you will consider it to be an educational resource—a reference to keep in your kitchen and guide you to good health.

Introduction

Part I consists of medical information by Paul Goldfinger, MD, FACC. He has had considerable experience in communicating medical topics to the public in his writings and lectures. He has reviewed the extensive medical literature regarding prevention. Although the book is intended for non-medical audiences, it is comprehensive and follows an "evidence based" framework. It respects the ability of lay people to understand these topics. He wants the reader to be knowledgeable and to know how doctors use research to inform their clinical decisions. The goal is to cover all aspects of prevention, although nutrition is stressed.

We will get into common clinical subjects such as heart attacks, high blood pressure, obesity, and high cholesterol. A wide variety of topics are covered including vitamin supplements, foods, medications, diets, therapeutic goals, exercise and many more.

Part II consists of heart-healthy recipes. A great deal of discussion and experimentation went into this section, because Eileen wanted to create delicious recipes that were easy to prepare, but they had to meet certain requirements, such as the central need to reduce fat content.

We were impressed by the potential value of fish as a heart healthy source of nutrients, and we wanted to educate readers regarding seafood preparation, so that was stressed in the recipes section. All these recipes have been developed and tested in our kitchen at home. Note that the food concepts presented in this book also provide valuable building blocks for a healthy weight loss plan.

Eileen begins with her Pantry section. She believes that certain ingredients need to be on hand, so that all you might require at the market would be the fresh components.

PART I:

Medical Information

By Paul Goldfinger, MD, FACC. Cardiologist

Definitions

Acute myocardial infarction ("heart attack" or "M.I.") is a serious and sudden event that results in injury and possibly permanent damage to heart muscle. An "M.I." occurs when a fatty plaque within the inner lining of a coronary artery becomes acutely disrupted. This results in clotting and obstruction of blood flow. It may have taken many years for the plaque to develop, and the narrowing often isn't severe prior to the event, but the acute injury to the plaque is what sets off a cascade of events within the artery which results in total blockage. There are impressive therapies available now for the treatment of acute myocardial infarction

Arteries are blood vessels that carry oxygen rich blood from the heart to organs and tissues throughout the body.

Atherosclerosis is a condition in which fatty deposits (*plaque*) build up inside the lining of arteries. The plaque deposits are complex and consist not only of fat, but also of scar tissue, calcium, inflammatory cells, and muscle tissue. The risk of acute complications, such as heart attack, is particularly great if the plaque consists of soft mushy fat deposits. If the buildup is severe enough to cause obstruction to blood flow, then symptoms will often develop. Atherosclerosis can involve the coronary arteries (causing heart attack or angina), the carotid arteries in the neck (causing stroke), or the leg arteries (causing pain with walking, i.e. claudication). Atherosclerosis can occur in other areas as well, such as the arteries to the kidneys or the intestines, causing kidney failure or abdominal pains. It takes many years for plaque to develop, and the earliest sign (the fatty streak) can be found in children as young as 10 years old. Plaque usually develops slowly and silently (i.e. without any symptoms), but early detection is often possible.

ATPIII is the Adult Treatment Panel of the National Cholesterol Education Program which provides guidelines for cholesterol management.

BMI (body mass index) is a number that tells you if you are overweight, obese or normal. It is obtained from a chart that utilizes your height and weight. These charts can be found on the internet (http://www.nhlbisupport.com/bmi/) Your doctor should have a copy of this chart. Twenty seven or less is a normal BMI. (NEJM 10/7/99). The lowest risk regarding weight is associated with a BMI of twenty five or less.

Cardiovascular refers to the entire system of heart and blood vessels (arteries and veins).

Cardiovascular disease *(CVD)* occurs when atherosclerosis compromises arterial blood flow and can involve the heart, brain, kidneys, legs and/or other vital areas of the body.

Cholesterol is a fatty substance found in all animal products, and the level in a person's blood relates to the amount of cholesterol ingested as well as to the body's ability to manufacture the substance in the liver. Genetic and dietary factors determine how much cholesterol is produced in the body. Vegetables do not contain cholesterol.

Coronary risk factors are the characteristics which make a person prone to develop coronary heart disease (CHD) and related cardiovascular disorders. They include high fat diets, high blood pressure, smoking, obesity, heredity, lack of exercise, diabetes, and abnormal blood cholesterol levels (especially high LDL and low HDL).

Coronary artery disease/coronary heart disease/atherosclerotic heart disease (CHD, CAD, or ASHD): This disease occurs when the coronary arteries (the arteries that supply the heart with oxygen) become partially or completely blocked by atherosclerotic plaque. A person with CHD may develop chest pains (angina), "heart attack" (myocardial infarction) or other complications, but it is also possible to feel fine and still have this condition (i.e. "silent" heart disease).

Complex carbohydrates are found in whole wheat flour, brown rice, potatoes, bran, legumes, soy, fruits and vegetables. These are "good carbs" because these foods contain substances that protect against cancer and heart disease.

CRP (C reactive protein). This blood protein is a "marker" for inflammation in the body. A blood test is available to measure CRP (high sensitivity CRP blood test), and a high reading has been correlated with risk for coronary disease. Increased risk is associated with levels above 2-3 mg/L. A level less than 1 mg/L is considered to be low risk.

HDL cholesterol (high density lipoprotein) is the "good cholesterol." This protein particle is responsible for "reverse transport" of cholesterol, which means that the cholesterol is carried away from the arteries and back to the liver for metabolism and removal from the body. This is the only lipid number that should be higher rather than lower. Levels that are low (i.e. under 40 mg/dl) are associated with increased heart attack risk, even if total cholesterol levels are normal.

Hyperlipidemia refers to elevations in blood lipids, such as hypercholesterolemia, which refers to high cholesterol levels, or hypertriglyceridema, which refers to high triglyceride levels.

Hypertension is a disease where the pressure in the arteries is too high (i.e. high blood pressure). The top number is the systolic, while the bottom is the diastolic.

Inflammation and/or infection in the body may be a risk factor, such as occurs with periodontal disease.

LDL cholesterol (low density lipoprotein) is the "bad cholesterol." LDL cholesterol becomes oxidized in the bloodstream, which means that it is chemically converted to a form that can stick to the interior lining of arteries and form plaque. It is the most important number in terms of risk, and that risk correlates with the degree of elevation. High levels relate mostly to dietary and genetic factors.

Lipids refer to the fatty components in the blood. If your doctor orders a "lipid panel" blood test, he will get total cholesterol, HDL, LDL, triglycerides and a risk ratio number. These results provide the basic information regarding lipid related risk. The test should be done with a 12-14 hour fast, although a simple cholesterol measurement does not have to be done fasting. The protein particles that carry fatty materials in the blood are called *lipoproteins.*

Metabolic Syndrome is a disorder which consists of a combination of characteristics that are associated with increased risk of cardiovascular problems. The syndrome includes abdominal obesity, abnormal lipids, high blood pressure, and diabetes/elevated insulin levels. The metabolic syndrome is associated with impaired lung function, mostly related to abdominal obesity. A French study found this condition to be more common in men with waist size of over 37 inches and, for women, 31 inches.

Monounsaturated fats (MUFA) such as olive oil and canola oil do not raise the levels of LDL cholesterol and may actually have some additional protective value. These fats, along with polyunsaturated fats, are often called "good fats."

Omega-3 fatty acids are polyunsaturated fats found in fish (i.e. fish oils). Fatty fish such as salmon, tuna and halibut are rich in these oils. There also are plant sources of omega-3's found in canola oil, nuts and many other plant sources. Feeding chickens high flax or algae diets has resulted in eggs rich in omega-3 fatty acids. Fish oils are also available in capsule form and in some margarine. Some processed foods, such as breads, are available fortified with omega-3 fatty acids.

Polyunsaturated fats (PUFA) are found in liquid vegetable oils including sunflower, cottonseed, safflower, corn, and soybean oils. These fats may be beneficial ("good fats") when used in modest amounts as part of a low fat diet. Unsaturated fatty acids do not raise LDL cholesterol levels.

Primary prevention refers to preventing disease in apparently healthy individuals.

Saturated fats are dietary fats, usually solid or semi-solid, derived mostly from animal sources such as red meats and dairy products, although some are derived from vegetable sources such as coconut and palm oil. The term "saturated" refers to the chemical composition of the fats. Saturated fats raise the levels of LDL cholesterol in the blood and are associated with increased risk for cardiovascular disease as well as being linked to colon, breast and prostate cancer.

Secondary prevention refers to reducing progression of disease in those who already are affected.

Simple carbohydrates such as sugar, alcohol, white flour, and white rice, are "bad carbs" that promote weight gain, conversion to fat and increased insulin levels.

Social issues seem to be associated with increased risk including low income, social isolation, low level of education, and stress/anxiety/depression.

Statins are drugs which reduce blood cholesterol levels by influencing the production of cholesterol within the liver.

Stroke is a general term (also called "CVA", or cerebrovascular accident) that describes brain injury resulting from either occluded brain arteries (usually due to atherosclerosis with thrombosis) or from brain hemorrhage. The risk of stroke correlates with the same "risk factors" as those associated with coronary heart disease, including hypertension, high cholesterol and smoking.

Thrombosis is clotting within a blood vessel. Thrombosis, occurring suddenly on top of atherosclerotic plaque in an artery, can cause acute complications such as heart attack or stroke.

Total cholesterol is the total concentration of cholesterol in the blood and consists of mostly LDL ("bad") cholesterol. The total also includes HDL ("good") cholesterol and a small amount that is carried with the triglycerides in the blood. The levels of total cholesterol correlate with risk of heart disease. In general, levels under 200 mg. are considered normal.

Trans-fats are artery clogging fats that form when liquid vegetable oils are converted into hard margarines. It also happens when vegetable oils are used for deep-frying. Trans-fats are found in stick margarines, doughnuts, French fries, shortenings, cookies, chips and crackers. Ingestion of trans-fats raises cholesterol and LDL levels and lowers HDL levels. Food manufacturers are now required to put trans-fats on their labels.

Triglycerides When elevated, these fatty particles are known to increase the risk of cardiovascular disease. Normal levels are under 130 mg. Individuals with very high levels (e.g. 500-2000 mg.) are also at risk for inflammation of the pancreas. Elevated triglycerides levels often occur with low HDL levels, and this combination is associated with a particularly high risk. Excess intake of carbohydrates, fats and alcohol contribute to high triglyceride levels.

Vascular refers to the blood vessels, particularly the arteries, which carry oxygen rich blood throughout the body. The functions of vital organs, including the heart and brain, depend on a good arterial blood flow. When arterial blood flow is inadequate due to narrowing of arteries, reduced tissue oxygen results. The medical term for this is ***ischemia.*** If arterial flow is completely obstructed, then tissue damage (***infarction***) may occur. The usual cause of such flow restriction is atherosclerosis (see below).

Concepts: Cholesterol Risks and Treatment

*I*t has been known for many years that elevated blood levels of cholesterol correlate with the risk of coronary heart disease (CHD). About 75% of patients with CHD have some type of lipid abnormality and most of these have elevated total and LDL cholesterol levels. The **Framingham Heart Study** showed that the risk of CHD was 3-5 times higher in men and women with total cholesterol levels of 300 mg. compared to 200 mg. Even for levels from 150-200 mg., the risk varies according to the degree of elevation.

Typical Americans have total cholesterol levels between 200-240 mg. and, although such levels are "normal" in the US, they are certainly not ideal and are high compared to many other parts of the world. In countries with average total cholesterol levels that are around 150 mg., heart attacks are rarely seen.

Most of the cholesterol in blood is found in the **LDL cholesterol** (low density lipoprotein) component of total cholesterol. The level of LDL cholesterol is the single most important number in assessing risk of atherosclerosis, because it is the component that promotes atherosclerotic buildup in arteries. The number relates to genetic and dietary factors. Diets that are high in saturated fats result in elevated LDL cholesterol levels.

There is strong evidence that low **HDL cholesterol** levels (less than 40 mg.) increase CHD risk, and that high (over 60 mg.) levels result in a reduced risk. Every 1 percent decrease in blood HDL is associated with a 2-3 percent increase in risk.

CHD can occur in people with "normal" cholesterol levels. The most common level among patients with coronary heart disease is 225 mg (Castelli. JACC. 1998). Since this number is fairly typical of many Americans, looking only at total cholesterol levels in "healthy" people is not enough to assess risk. We now know that measuring both LDL and HDL cholesterol levels together can more accurately evaluate risk. If one divides the total cholesterol by the HDL you get a ***risk ratio***, which is, according to the Framingham Heart Study, the "best predictor of coronary artery disease". High triglycerides also pose a risk, especially if coupled with a low HDL level.

Normalizing abnormal cholesterol levels can improve risk. (See later sections on therapy). LDL levels can be lowered dramatically with diet and drugs. The most difficult therapeutic task in lipid therapy is raising the HDL level. HDL cholesterol increases of only 6% have been associated with significant reductions in coronary morbidity and mortality in patients with low HDL levels. (Rader, Medscape 6/04). For raising HDL levels, regular aerobic exercise can help, as can stopping smoking and losing weight. Fish oils have been reported to raise HDL levels by about 8%. Drug therapy for treating low HDL is discussed later.

Research is ongoing as to how cholesterol lowering actually works. It appears that much of the benefit has to do with alterations in the fatty deposits that build up inside arteries. Aggressive lowering of serum cholesterol helps to remove these fatty deposits within the plaque, thus creating a more stable situation within the artery, even if the degree of narrowing remains unchanged. Some of the benefits occur soon after starting cholesterol drugs and seem to be related to mechanisms such as altered blood clotting and reduced arterial spasm. Such early benefits are independent of cholesterol lowering, and physicians have begun initiating cholesterol-lowering medications very early during an acute event, such as starting statin drugs in the coronary care unit after a heart attack.

Concepts: Nutrition in Preventing Heart Disease

*I*n America, we eat too much junk food, processed food, and saturated fat; and too little vegetables, fruits and whole grains. Our portion sizes are too large, and our people are among the fattest in the world. Atherosclerosis prevention requires a multifaceted approach that aims to treat multiple risk factors, but the nutrition aspects are stressed in this book.

In general, a **heart healthy diet** focuses on reduction of animal fats, so dietary fat reduction is a key element in the nutritional approach to preventing heart disease. But there are many other related nutritional specifics which will be discussed, including fresh fruits, vegetables, fiber, nuts, fish, good oils, legumes and whole grains, among others. These types of healthy foods offer benefits in the prevention of stroke, diabetes, hypertension, cancer and heart disease and they are important components in weight reduction, especially if coupled with portion and caloric control. Other benefits to be obtained from heart-healthy eating include favorable influences on insulin and sugar levels, colon health, and brain function.

Most people who believe that they are on a low fat diet are actually on a "less fat diet" and could do much better in terms of reducing their intake of fats. Many low fat diets stipulate that 30% of calories be derived from fat. But some diets are much stricter in terms of fat restriction, with fat limits down to 10-15% of calories. (*Archives of Internal Medicine*, July 10, 2006). Dr. Dean Ornish is famous for his extremely low fat diets.

It is important to realize that most low fat diets generally lower cholesterol levels by only modest amounts (usually in the 10-20% range). The amount of cholesterol lowering that occurs with diet is quite variable, depending largely on genetic factors and patient compliance. Diets form the foundation of efforts to correct abnormal blood lipids, but often medications must be added in order to achieve excellent results.

Low fat diets, by definition, contain reduced fats, but the type of fat that one consumes is an important concern. Recent research suggests that the type of dietary fat may be more important than the amount of total fat. Unsaturated fats ("good fats") do not cause LDL levels to go up. Saturated fats ("bad fats") are usually derived from animal products such as red meats and dairy products. They cause LDL cholesterol levels to go up and then to become deposited in arteries. A diet low in saturated fats eliminates most meat, cheese, ice cream, whole and 2% milk, butter, cakes and pastries. If you eat meat, it should be low in fat, such as poultry and fish. If you have some red meat in your diet, then it should be very lean. Some red meats are particularly lean, including venison, ostrich and buffalo.

All recommended heart-healthy diets restrict cholesterol intake. Foods with saturated fats are usually high in cholesterol, but there are some foods such as eggs, lobster and shrimp, which are low in fat but high in cholesterol. These foods can be acceptable in a heart healthy diet, but in limited amounts.

The fat grams that you do consume should be mostly of vegetable origin and should be unsaturated (either monounsaturated as in olive and canola oil or polyunsaturated as in some vegetable oil margarines or liquid oils such as corn or safflower). Fish contain beneficial fish oils. Unsaturated fats can be used to substitute for saturated fats, but they do not contain fewer calories.

Diets for Heart Health

There are a variety of heart healthy diets available, and there are debates about which are best. All good heart healthy diets restrict saturated fats and encourage maintaining an ideal weight. Some experts such as Dr. William Castelli of Framingham believe that the best approach is to adopt a *vegetarian diet.*

However, besides becoming a vegetarian, it appears that a *Mediterranean type diet* is the most sensible choice for prevention. You can follow the basic principles as discussed below and design a style of eating that is customized to your requirements or you can follow one of the specific diets noted below.

To accomplish your dietary goals, you must stick to the regimen, allowing only rare exceptions. Remember that a coronary problem can progress under the surface and strike without warning. *Do not refer to yourself as being on a diet. Instead you must view this as a lifestyle change* that will govern how you eat forever. Instead of following strict diet rules which are hard to maintain, you can adapt the principles of heart healthy-eating into your own personal method. If you learn how to eat and how to prepare foods properly at home, you will find that this approach can be enjoyable and you will not feel deprived. (See part II of this book regarding food preparation).

If you want a specific diet, *The American Heart Association* and the *National Cholesterol Education Program* diets are very similar, although the terminology is confusing. These diets are variously called Step 1, Step 2 or TLC, and you can read the details at the web sites. Basically, they call for reduction in total and saturated dietary fat to less than 30% of total energy intake. They also stress whole grains, fiber, fruits and vegetables. In my opinion, individuals with known heart disease should consume less than 20% of total calories from fat and little or no calories from saturated fat. The rest of one's daily energy requirement (i.e. 70% or less of calories) will come from carbohydrates (preferably complex carbs) and proteins. *Most of what you eat should be derived from plants.*

"Mediterranean diets" have been linked to reduced risk due to the fact that they contain monounsaturated fats from olive oil, plus fruits, whole grains, fiber, vegetables, garlic, nuts, legumes, red wine, poultry, and ocean fish. This diet is not necessarily low in fat, but the fats consumed are unsaturated "good fats". There are quite a few countries bordering the Mediterranean, and there is some variation in their diets. Avoid the ones that contain a lot of pork, cheese, butter, milk and beef. Make believe you are a fisherman from Sicily or Crete.

A fascinating trial from France (*Lyon Diet Heart Study. Circulation.*1999) found that a modified "Mediterranean diet" is cardioprotective and will significantly reduce the risk of cardiac death and recurrent heart attacks. The difference between the traditional Mediterranean diet and the one used in the French study is that the oil used in the Lyon trial was canola oil enriched with omega-3 fatty acids (as in fish oils) instead of olive oil. What is curious about these two diets is that they did not lower serum cholesterol levels, so it seems that the oils used in these diets protect the arteries in ways other than cholesterol lowering.

Many experts believe that the monounsaturated composition of olive oil is protective, and that extra virgin olive oil seems to have more protective qualities than refined olive oil, due to greater amounts of antioxidant components. (J. of Nutrition.1999) However, before you decide to use unlimited amounts of olive or canola oil, remember that fats of all kinds are high in calories and will promote weight gain. A tablespoon of olive oil has the same 12 grams of fat (110 cal.) as a tablespoon of butter, so even though olive oil is healthier than butter, it is no less fattening. Manufacturers of new margarines, like Smart Balance®, say that their "buttery spreads" have 80 calories per serving (1 tbsp), so there may be a small advantage there, and they use a blend of "good oils" including olive, canola and soy, with some preparations also containing fish oil and plant sterols.

Other low fat diets: There are some low fat diets that are stricter than the AHA (*e.g. Ornish*), but following these diets is difficult for most individuals. Also, one sees a substantial drop in HDL ("good") cholesterol, and the significance of this is uncertain.

Dr Ornish's *Lifestyle Heart Trial* has reported a 5-year follow-up in his patients treated with a very strict low fat diet, exercise, stress management and psychosocial support. He uses no drugs. He has shown that his patients had excellent cholesterol blood levels, lower complications (such as chest pains) and small amounts of plaque regression compared to those treated with less vigorous diets. (*JAMA* 280:2001). He says that his patients have success in terms of weight control and regression of coronary plaque because they keep their fat intake far below the 30% suggested by the AHA and they are strict in controlling portion size and intake of simple carbs. Dr. Ornish's various books are all excellent, especially "Eat More, Weigh Less."

The **DASH diet** is a balanced 2000-calorie diet that is a good compromise between the very low fat diets and the American Heart Association diet. It has been recommended by the Joint National Committee on Prevention, Detection, Evaluation, and Treatment of High Blood Pressure (NIH publication # 98-4080). DASH stands for "Dietary Approaches to Stop Hypertension," a clinical trial that evaluated the management of high blood pressure. The diet was recommended for patients with hypertension, but it is also beneficial in efforts to prevent heart disease and cancer. DASH supplies 27% of calories from fat (mostly unsaturated) and includes a lot of fruits, vegetables, grains, nuts, seeds, beans as well as small amounts of unsaturated oil such as found in salad dressing, peanut butter and mayonnaise. The DASH diet recommends low fat dairy products such as yogurt as well as increased intake of calcium, potassium and magnesium.

Diets for Losing Weight

A ccording to Dr. K. Brownell, the director of the Rudd Center of Food Policy and Obesity at Yale, people spend a great deal of money on special diets for weight loss, but "the truth is that success depends not so much on what diet plan you choose or what program you join. What matters most is your level of motivation and your willingness to change."

Most popular diets result in an average weight loss after two years of nine pounds. The trend now is to encourage people to forget about rigid diets and, instead, to focus on portion size, calories, exercise and psychological factors such as motivation. Increased vegetable intake is encouraged, as is reduction in dietary fat. You can view this article by Lesley Alderman at *NYTimes.com*, July 4, 2009 and *The Washington Post*, Feb 4, 2010.

The **Atkins diet** for weight reduction is high in fats and low in carbohydrates. With this diet, adherents are encouraged to eat red meat, bacon, eggs and other proteins that are high in saturated fat. Although such a diet can help people lose weight, it is the carbohydrate restriction that seems to be the most important element. Patients on the Atkins diet do get a drop in total cholesterol due to reduced triglycerides, but the bad LDL cholesterol levels do not drop. Although the HDL levels may rise with Atkins, this is not a positive result, according to Dr Dean Ornish. He says, "I think that (the Atkins diet) is dangerous to your health." He says that "the high fat, high protein content increases the risk of heart disease, diabetes, hypertension, breast/prostate/colon cancer and most of the chronic degenerative diseases" (These quotes are from a *PBS* interview that Dr Ornish gave in 2004). According to Gerald Reuven, MD, professor of medicine at Stanford, "The Atkins diet is dangerous..." (*Nutrition Action Health Letter,* March 2000).

The best approach is to modify the Atkins diet by reducing saturated fat but continuing the carbohydrate restriction. Eliminate bread and pasta. Fill up on vegetables, low fat meats/fish, legumes, fruits, and nonfat dairy products. Low saturated fat diets have been proven to prevent heart disease, whereas the Atkins diet is unproved and may be hazardous in terms of coronary risk. Remember that one can gain weight with a heart healthy diet if calories are not limited.

See the section on obesity in the "Special Patient Populations" section on pages 28 and 29."

Nutrition Issues Regarding Certain Foods

ish: The **omega-3 polyunsaturated fatty acids ("fish oils")** derived from eating fish are called EPA and DHA. There is evidence to suggest that these oils will help prevent heart disease, stroke and sudden death. Populations that eat a lot of fish, such as the Inuit Eskimos, have low cholesterol levels and low risk of heart attacks and sudden death. In one trial where people ate at least 8.75 ounces (about ½ pound) of fish per week, there was a 35% reduced risk of heart attacks. Fish oils lower triglycerides and may raise HDL levels. They do not have much effect on LDL cholesterol levels. Fatty fish have especially high levels of omega-3's.

Omega-3 fatty acids also lower high blood pressure and have favorable effects on clotting and heart rhythm. Eating fish not only helps prevents disease, but it is a nutritious high protein food with many vitamins and minerals. There is concern about high mercury content in some fish.

Other sources of omega-3 fatty acids include cashew nuts, soybeans, canola oil and English walnuts. Omega-3 fatty acids are also found in margarines such as Smart Balance Regular with flax oil.

We recommend having fish frequently, but it must be cooked by grilling, broiling, poaching, or baking. Large fish like tuna pose a risk because of mercury contamination. If the fish is sautéed, do it in a Teflon coated pan with a spray of olive oil or a little Benecol®. Most fish consumed in this country is fried, and this is undesirable. See discussion of fish oil supplements below.

Shellfish such as lobster and shrimp are high in cholesterol but are also rich in fish oils and can be included in this regimen. I believe a limited amount of shrimp and lobster is acceptable. (But cook it "low fat" and don't dunk it in butter!—use cocktail sauce or melt some "regular" Benecol® or Heart Smart ® margarine)

Fiber: Adequate amounts of fiber can reduce the risk of heart disease, high cholesterol levels, colon cancer, recurrent diverticulitis, gallstones, varicose veins and obesity. Soluble (viscous) fiber, taken as 5-10 grams per day can lower LDL cholesterol levels by about 5%.

Soluble fiber includes oats, pectin, barley, pectin rich fruit, psyllium (Metamucil®) and beans. Insoluble fiber does not reduce cholesterol levels.

Nutritionists usually recommend 25-30 grams of fiber (soluble and insoluble) per day, taken by eating whole grains (e.g. oats), fruits, vegetables, beans and nuts. Most Americans consume less than half the recommended amount.

A high fiber cereal (such as bran or Cheerios®) is a good source. Choose cereals that offer at least three grams of fiber per bowl. Half a grapefruit provides six grams of fiber, while an apple provides five. All fruits contain fiber.

Eggs: The egg industry says that eating eggs is healthy, because eggs contain no fat and do not raise cholesterol levels. The American Heart Association disagrees, pointing out that each egg yolk contains 300 mg. of cholesterol, and research trials have shown that eating cholesterol promotes heart disease, even if the cholesterol levels do not rise (*Nutrition Action Healthletter* July 1997). According to Jeremiah Stamler, a world expert on prevention, eggs do raise total and bad (LDL) cholesterol levels. The AHA recommends that individuals eat no more than four egg yolks per week. Other experts advocate reducing egg intake to only one or two eggs per week (JAMA 4/21/99).

Egg substitutes (e.g. "Eggbeaters"®) are an excellent way to enjoy eggs without the fat, but you need to prepare them with just a light spray of monounsaturated oil in the pan. Egg dishes can also be made with egg whites, since egg whites contain no cholesterol.

Chocolate contains saturated fats (especially if milk is added) and traditionally is forbidden in low fat diets, but dark chocolate also contains flavenoids, which are chemicals that can relax blood vessels and reduce the tendency of blood to clot. Flavenoids are also potent antioxidants and are found in red wine, cherries, apricots, apples and green tea. Some studies suggest a reduced cardiovascular risk with increased flavenoid intake. There may be some health benefits from chocolate, but the research so far is inconclusive. Chocolate is fattening and has too much fat. It is best to only eat small amounts.

Soy contains high quality protein and essential fatty acids and can be a good replacement for animal food products. Soy can produce small reductions in LDL levels. Studies suggest that cardiac protection may occur with 25-30 grams of soy protein per day.

Nuts: A number of trials suggest a protective benefit of a small amount of nuts per day. Nuts contain unsaturated fat, usually of the monounsaturated and omega 3 fatty acid types. A recent analysis of 34,000 Seventh Day Adventists found a fairly powerful reduction in risk by eating nuts about 5 times per week. (*Archives of Internal Medicine* 10/97). In the Nurses Health study of over 86,000 women, eating more than 5 ounces of nuts per week resulted in a reduced risk of fatal and nonfatal heart disease. (*British Med. J.* Nov, 1998)

Different kinds of nuts have different nutrient compositions. Walnuts are considered the most heart healthy because they contain alpha-linolenic acid, which is similar to the omega-3 fatty acids found in fish oil. Cashews are a good source of monounsaturated fats. Watch out for nuts that are packed with salt and do not eat coconuts because they are high in saturated fat. Remember that nuts are fattening (usually 160-190 calories per ounce), however at least one study showed that a modest regular consumption of nuts does not cause extra weight gain.

Alcohol: Heavy consumption of alcohol increases the risk of dying, but small amounts of alcohol seem to offer some protection against coronary disease. In the Physicians Health Study (*Lancet* 1998), 5,358 male physicians who had a history of heart attack were questioned as to alcohol intake. During a 5-year follow-up, small amounts of alcohol (from 2-4 drinks per week up to one drink per day) resulted in a reduction in cardiovascular mortality risk. Taking more than that resulted in less benefit. The benefits of alcohol are believed to relate to raising HDL levels, inhibiting LDL oxidation, and reducing blood clotting.

Many experts believe that 1-2 glasses of ***red wine*** per day may offer better protection than other forms of alcohol. Red wine contains resveratrol, a substance that may be protective, but red wine also contains flavenoids, which are antioxidant substances. Grape skins or grape juice may be of value, but it is not established that grape juice is just as effective as red wine in prevention. Alcohol may give red wine the edge over grape juice. ATPIII suggests no more than two drinks per day for men and no more than one drink per day for women. A drink is 5 ounces of wine. Individuals with a history of alcohol or drug dependency should not use alcohol in any form.

Black and green teas contain flavenoids that may protect the heart.

The best study on tea is from Holland (*Archives Int. Med.* Oct 11, 1999), which found that black tea was associated with less atherosclerotic plaque in the aorta (the body's main artery), but other studies show no protective benefit. Adding milk to your tea may reduce the benefits. Other trials suggest that 3-4 cups of tea per day may protect against heart attacks and strokes. These claims should not be considered to be proven.

Coffee confers no protection, and some studies in the past have suggested an increased risk with coffee. If coffee is boiled, as in Europe, it can raise cholesterol levels, but if filtered, as in the U.S., it does not. In addition, some studies suggest a health benefit of coffee in lowering risk of gall bladder disease and colon cancer. A recent trial suggested that coffee can protect against Alzheimer's disease. Caffeine and/or flavenoids seem to be the beneficial ingredients.

Some individuals are sensitive to the *caffeine* in coffee and can experience heart palpitations, anxiety and insomnia. It is not true that all heart patients need to eliminate caffeine, but you should check with your doctor. Watch for hidden sources of caffeine such as colas and dark chocolate. Tea has 50 mg, while coffee has 135 mg of caffeine per 8 oz. cup. Colas contain 37-45 mg in 12 oz, while dark chocolate has 30 mg in a 1 ½ ounce bar.

Salt consists of sodium and chloride. The average *sodium* intake for healthy adults is 2,400 mg (2.4 grams) which is the same as 4,800 mg of sodium chloride (i.e. salt). This amounts to about one teaspoon of salt each day. Reading labels is important, because processed foods (e.g. canned soups) often contain excess salt.

Certain patients require severe restriction of salt, such as those with fluid retention from various causes. However, there is reason to believe that everyone should avoid excessive salt intake, especially if you have high blood pressure. There is some controversy regarding dietary salt, so you should discuss your salt intake with your doctor.

Nutrition Issues Regarding Food Supplements

ish oil supplements: Capsules containing fish oils may offer the benefits of omega-3 fatty acids, but most of the evidence of benefit was obtained from studying people who ate fish frequently. Taking fish oil capsules may reduce the risk of heart attacks and other complications, but the evidence is still incomplete. One cannot assume that fish oil capsules will confer the same protection as eating fish. On the other hand, the Italian *GISSI Trial* found a moderate reduction in cardiac risk with fish oil supplements.

Diarrhea and esophageal reflux are common side effects of fish oil supplements, and they also can cause some fishy burping or fishy breath. There may be a risk of bleeding, as well as toxicity from impurities such as mercury. Supplements must be properly purified, so they must be obtained from reputable sources. A recent evaluation of 41 common fish oil products found that none were contaminated with mercury or PCB's. Your pharmacist can offer some advice in this regard, but do not take fish oils without discussing the decision with your physician.

Vitamins used to be recommended as preventive therapy due to their anti-oxidant actions. In recent years, however, large trials have shown no benefit with vitamins, so these supplements can no longer be considered part of a prevention regimen. This conclusion does not apply to vitamins found in fruits and vegetables. For individuals who have a poor diet, they could become deficient in certain vitamins. They should be on a daily vitamin supplement. There is a blood test to detect vitamin deficiencies. Some vitamin and herbal supplements can interfere with cardiac medications (as can grapefruit juice), so check with your doctor.

Vitamin E: Prior trials have suggested that vitamin E (alpha tocopherol), 75 to 400 units per day can reduce the risk of heart attacks and stroke, but a recent large study (HOPE Trial; *New England Journal*. 2000 Jan.) found no value for Vitamin E in thousands of heart attack survivors. In a Harvard trial of over 40,000 male physicians, vitamin intake did not prevent stroke. (*Annals of Int. Med.* 6/15/99)

The vitamins studied included Vitamin E, C, and beta-carotene. In an Italian study of over 11,000 heart attack survivors, vitamin E was of no value. (*Lancet.* 8/7/99; GISSI Trial). There are some worrisome results which found that over 400 IU per day of vitamin E could increase the risk of death. (*NY Times*, March 24, 2009). There are similar concerns about increased risk with vitamin A supplements.

Beta-carotene is an antioxidant which may be dangerous in smokers and should not be taken in high dosage according to a trial from Finland. There is no good evidence that it is protective, and there is a suggestion that beta carotene may be carcinogenic.

Vitamin C (ascorbic acid) is a popular supplement, but the evidence of benefit is "inconclusive" according to the *Harvard Men's Health Watch*. A trial from the University of Southern California described a possible harmful effect of Vitamin C, and the scientists who did the study said that people who take vitamin C should stop. (*Internal Med. News* May 2000).

Vitamin D is important for bone health, but recent research shows that many Americans are deficient, and deficiencies are linked to heart disease, heart failure and hypertension in addition to many other problems. There is evidence that Vitamin D therapy can be protective against heart disease, although more studies are necessary. The typical recommended dose is 400-1000 units per day, although more research is needed regarding dosing. Many doctors urge their patients to undergo blood testing for vitamin D levels. If the level is low, they often order supplements, but the value of this approach is controversial.

Niacin (Vit. B3) can lower LDL cholesterol levels and can substantially raise HDL cholesterol levels, but it must be used in high dosage and only under a physician's supervision. It is the best drug for raising HDL.

Selenium is an antioxidant and is promoted as a way to prevent heart disease and cancer. A prior study showed that 200 micrograms per day could reduce the risk of prostate, colon and lung cancers. However, selenium can be obtained through the diet in the form of vegetables, whole grains, fish, dairy products and meat. Discuss the use of this and other supplements with your physician.

Chinese red yeast rice: This diet supplement is a fermented product of rice on which red yeast has been grown. It contains natural statins (such as are found in cholesterol lowering drugs). It can reduce cholesterol and triglycerides, but the active ingredient and the side effects are similar to those of the statin drugs (*Am. J. of Clinical Nutrition.* 1999; 69:231). A 2009 trial in the *Annals of Internal Medicine* showed that lowering LDL cholesterol can be significant with this dietary supplement and that it might be useful in patients who cannot tolerate statins. The trial was small, and further study is required. In addition, there is no pharmaceutical grade version of this substance available and no approval by the FDA, so it is best to avoid this supplement and to discuss it with your doctor.

Coenzyme Q10 is an antioxidant similar to Vitamin E. It occurs naturally in food and is sold in health food stores and online. Claims have been made for benefits in prevention and treatment, but the evidence so far does not support its long-term use.

Garlic: This tasty ingredient for great recipes is said to reduce cholesterol, but some research suggests otherwise. Garlic also has been associated with reduced blood clotting and lowered blood pressure. For individuals on blood thinners like Coumadin, garlic can increase the risk of bleeding. At present the evidence does not support using garlic supplements for prevention. ATPIII also does not recommend herbal or botanical dietary supplements of any other kind, including grapeseed extract, ginseng, or cranberry.

Homocysteine is an amino acid which is found in everyone's blood. However, if the blood levels are high (over 15 mmol/L), the risk of atherosclerosis is increased. Normal blood levels are about 9-15mmol/L. The goal is to have a level of 9-10. *Folic acid* and B vitamins can bring the number down, and some physicians prescribe 1-2 mg of folic acid per day to lower homocysteine. Recent trials, however, have failed to show that treating homocysteine will reduce cardiac risk.

Plant stanols/sterols are naturally occurring substances, sometimes called phytonutrients, which can lower LDL cholesterol levels by 7-14%. They are obtained from pine trees or soy beans and they work by blocking cholesterol absorption in the intestines. Stanols/sterols are available in margarines such as Benecol®, or in combination with aspirin or vitamins, or alone. They reduce LDL cholesterol levels and have no effect on HDL. The ATPIII guidelines say that one needs 2 grams of stanols/sterols per day to reduce LDL cholesterol. It is recommended that phytonutrients be taken about 15 minutes before eating. One theoretical concern is that they may do very little when someone is on a strict low fat diet and they may block absorption of good oils. Discuss their use with your physician, especially if you are already on cholesterol medication

Dietary Tips

You must be extremely careful in **restaurants**. It is always difficult to be sure how much fat and calories you are getting in a restaurant. Do not hesitate to ask the waiter or chef about the ingredients in their dishes. Good restaurants will adapt to your needs. Note that chefs like to slip butter and salt into their dishes to give flavor, and you may never guess it from the menu description.

Stay away from Chinese restaurants, steak houses and fast food places. A large hamburger with onion rings contains 1,550 calories and 101 grams of fat. A tuna salad sandwich has 720 calories and 43 grams of fat. Salads are not low calorie if they are covered with fatty dressings.

Home cooked meals, where you know the ingredients, are the way to go most of the time, but someone at home needs to learn how to cook. Dr. Castelli from the Framingham Trial says that most families eat the same things week after week (e.g. meat loaf every Thursday). He says that people need to learn some new recipes to replace the old ones.

Take advantage of the **nonfat and low fat products** that are now available. These items make it easier to adhere to a low fat regimen. Home cooking will enable you to use fresh ingredients and to avoid processed foods which contain chemicals that might be harmful. Read Michael Pollan's book "*The Omnivore's Dilemma*" about the food industry. He says not to eat anything which your grandmother would not recognize as food. Make low fat recipes at home that will satisfy the craving for meat (e.g. meatballs made of ground white meat turkey). Part II of this book will help you find such recipes.

Be careful of "low fat" products that actually have more fat than you should be taking. Watch out for items that say "no cholesterol". These foods, such as potato chips, may have no cholesterol, but they still can be very high in fat. Watch out for foods that are labeled "vegetarian" but may contain a lot of fat. Note also that many fat free foods have as many calories as their full fat counterparts. For example, one ounce of fat free pretzels contains as many calories (110) as the regular type, so read the labels for calories as well as fats.

Eating *protein* will aid in weight control, although Dr. Ornish says that high protein intake promotes heart disease and cancer. Good sources of protein include poultry, fish, soy products (e.g. tofu), legumes, skim milk, low fat cottage cheese, nonfat cheeses, and frozen yogurt. If you are having meat, use the reduced fat variety and try to keep the amount per portion down to 4 ounces (about as much as you can fit in the palm of your hand). Low fat dairy products also provide much needed calcium, especially for older individuals who are in danger of bone loss.

Avoid large amounts of *simple carbohydrates,* such as pastas and white bread. These items can promote weight gain, raise triglyceride levels and lower the levels of good (HDL) cholesterol. Try to eliminate sugar and other refined sweeteners. Be aware that some of the nonfat or low fat products contain a great deal of sugar. *Complex carbohydrates* such as in beans, fruits, and starches are preferable to those derived from sugar. Most grain consumed in the US is refined, but whole grains are healthier and may be beneficial by reducing blood clotting and inflammation. Try to switch to a breakfast cereal containing whole grains, and use breads made with whole grains such as whole wheat. Frequent consumption of dried beans and peas has been found to produce a reduced cardiovascular risk (*Internal Medicine News.* May 2000)

Non-fat soup stocks such as Pritikin® chicken broth or vegetable broth help to add flavor to your non-fat meals. If you buy processed foods such as canned soups, read the labels for sodium content. Keep your sodium intake to fewer than 2000 mg per day (or less if you are on a strict low salt diet). If the label gives the amount of salt in grams, note that the sodium content is about half of that, and one gram (gm) is the same as 1000 milligrams (mg).

Salads are fine for this program, but you must not have bacon bits, cheese or meat in the salad, unless they are the nonfat type. Two tablespoons of salad dressing is likely to contain 10-20 grams of fat from oil. According to the CSPI, "The average woman aged 19-50 gets more fat from salad dressing than from any other food". (*Nutrition Action Health Letter* July 1997) Use only low fat dressings or just a small amount of olive oil and vinegar.

Other Prevention Issues

M*ental Health*: It has been known for some time that stress, anxiety, social isolation and hostility/anger may increase the risk of heart disease. Now there is evidence that ***depression*** is also a "potent" risk factor for coronary disease and has been linked to increased risk of stroke, hypertension and carotid artery disease. (*Harvard Men's Health Watch*, Nov. 1999). These observations have been made in both men and women. Similarly, for those who have had heart attacks, the risk of dying during the 6-12 months after the attack is greater in those with depression, and the adverse risk can extend for years later. Research is trying to determine if psychiatric drugs such as Prozac can make a difference in the risk after a heart attack. It should be noted that not all experts agree regarding the role of psychological factors in causing coronary heart disease. A study from Walter Reed Medical Center found no relationship between depression, anxiety, hostility and stress in promoting coronary artery disease (*NEJM*,11/2/2000)

Exercise: Physical inactivity is associated with increased risk for CHD and is listed by ATPIII as a major risk factor. Increased physical activity is associated with a reduced risk for CHD. Advantages of exercise include a lower risk of diabetes, less tendency for blood to clot, improved lipids including higher HDL levels, improved sleep patterns, and reduced anxiety and depression. Other benefits reported include reduced colon cancer, reduced gallstones, reduced arthritis symptoms, lower blood pressure, less prostate enlargement and less osteoporosis (weak bones in the elderly).

A regular aerobic exercise program is a necessary adjunct to a good diet. It is very difficult to lose weight without exercise, but don't be discouraged if the weight loss is slow. Exercise does not burn a lot of calories. Walking or running a mile will burn only about 100 calories, but exercise improves fitness and thus allows you to do more exercise and burn more calories. Also, the calories that are burned are more likely to be from fat than from carbohydrates, and the ability to keep weight off after losing is easier with regular exercise.

The amount of exercise necessary is controversial; however, a brisk walk 4-5 times per week can offer some protection. In the Nurses Health Study from Harvard, women who regularly engage in brisk walking reduced their risk of heart disease to the same degree as women who engaged in vigorous exercise. Some studies suggest that strenuous efforts are probably better.

An exercise prescription based on your heart rate is a good technique for judging how hard to exercise, and your doctor can give you advice about this. Pulse monitors, (e.g. by Polar© at polarusa.com) are available in sporting goods stores. If you are healthy, you can get a fitness evaluation at the local YMCA and receive advice regarding an exercise program, or, if there are concerns about coronary risk, a formal exercise stress test ordered by your physician would be appropriate. The Center for Disease Control suggests that people should get at least 30 minutes of moderate activity on most, or preferably all, days of the week.

If someone has underlying heart disease, vigorous physical exercise can be risky, especially if the patient is not accustomed to regular exercise. Sometimes people who have no awareness that they have heart trouble can be at risk for complications during exercise. Individuals with heart disease or who are at risk for heart disease should speak to their doctors before engaging in strenuous forms of exercise. According to Barry Maron, MD, an expert on the subject of cardiac events during exercise, "The balance of the evidence supports the value and importance of participation in regular exercise regimens (NEJM.11/9/2000).

Smoking: ATPIII says that cigarette smoking is a strong, independent risk factor for CHD. Even smoking one cigarette per day increases the risk of cardiovascular disease, although the risk does correlate with the amount smoked. Second hand smoke is now known to increase risk as well. Cigar/pipe smoking also carries an increased risk, even though cigar/pipe smokers do not inhale. As many as 30% of US deaths may be related to cigarette smoking. (Circulation. 1997:3243). People who quit smoking tend to gain about 10-15 lbs, but that can be offset by exercise and diet. Stopping smoking reduces the risk of CVD events, and that decline in risk, according to ATPIII, begins within months after quitting.

Inflammation or infection: It has been found that traditional risk factors can estimate risk of cardiovascular disease in only about 50-60% of the population. Scientists are looking for other factors that might improve the ability to predict who might be a candidate for atherosclerosis. It has been found recently that certain blood tests which measure inflammation/infection in the body correlate with risk.

The most common of these tests is called "high sensitivity C reactive protein" or CRP. The Jupiter Trial found that treating apparently healthy people with normal LDL cholesterol levels and high CRP levels, using a statin drug (rosuvastatin), resulted in reduced risk of coronary disease events. (*Circulation* 2003; 108:2292.) In 2009, the Jupiter Trial showed that treatment also reduced the risk of stroke.

The most recent research has found that treating high CRP levels is not supported by large population studies, but the test can still be used to identify high risk patients and to choose which persons with normal cholesterol levels might be treated with statin drugs.

Another intriguing related idea is that **poor oral hygiene** can be a factor in causing atherosclerosis. The concept hasn't been fully explored, but it is reasonable to ask patients with known coronary heart disease and those with high risk for CVD to maintain good oral hygiene and have routine dental cleanings, perhaps every 3-4 months. Rinsing with Listerine® twice per day, 30 seconds minimum per rinse, is a practical daily approach along with brushing and flossing.

Special Patient Populations

*P*atients with established CHD have a risk of recurrent myocardial infarction and CHD death of 20% over 10 years. Secondary prevention in this group requires very aggressive methods, with reduction in LDL levels being the most important variable. See below for discussion of treatment goals for LDL reduction. Of course every technique for reducing risk should be adopted.

Obesity has been upgraded to a "major" risk factor for heart disease by the American Heart Association. (Circulation.1999; 97:2099). The official statement said, "Obesity is a chronic disease, just like high blood pressure or high cholesterol. Its causes are a complex, individualized combination of genetics, behavior and lifestyle that we are just now beginning to understand".

The latest way to judge body weight is by checking your "*body mass index*." You look up your height and weight on a chart, and then a number is revealed called the BMI. Over 27 is considered overweight. Obesity is over 30. BMI charts are available on the internet. http://nhlbisupport.com/BMI/. It is estimated that 28% of men and 33% of women age 20-74 are obese, but these numbers continue to rise.

Obesity is directly related to high cholesterol levels, high blood pressure, high triglycerides, excess insulin, excess clotting factors, low levels of "good cholesterol", and increased mortality risk from cardiovascular disease, congestive heart failure, diabetes and hypertension. (*Cardiology Review.* 1999, August). Obesity also increases the risk of recurrent coronary disease after bypass surgery.

Research has shown that even modest weight reduction of 5-10% of body weight can reduce high blood pressure, total cholesterol, and cardiac risk. There is a tendency to gain weight as one ages due to lower metabolic rates and reduced physical activity. Muscle mass tends to decrease while fat cells increase. Since fat cells burn fewer calories than muscle cells, weight gain occurs. Exercise can help counteract this gain by burning more calories and, through strength training, by building up muscle.

Weight reduction requires that you count calories and exercise. Buy a kitchen scale to weigh your food. Pay close attention to portion size. In some families or restaurants, a serving may contain 2 or 3 portions. If someone hands you a plate of food, you should consider eating only part of it.

Reducing calories is still a valid concept for weight control. Counting fat calories is particularly important since fats contain more calories than carbs or proteins. Since each gram of fat contains 9 calories, you can count fat grams (read it on a food label) and multiply by nine to figure out how many calories in your diet are derived from fat. One tablespoon of oil contains 14 grams of fat (i.e. 126 calories.) Carbohydrates and proteins contain four calories per gram.

For example, if you are on a 2000-calorie AHA diet, you can have 600 calories (30% of total calories) from fat per day (i.e. 67 grams of fat per day; 600 divided by 9). The AHA specifically suggests that less than 7% of total calories should come from saturated fats, so most of the fat grams that you ingest should come from unsaturated or polyunsaturated food sources, preferably from plants.

Studies show that weight reduction can occur to about the same degree with the Mediterranean, Atkins or low fat diets, provided that calorie intakes are reduced. (NEJM 360:859-873, 2009)

Hypertension: High blood pressure is a major risk factor for cardiovascular diseases. It is a common disorder that usually has a genetic basis and thus tends to run in families. It is estimated that about fifty million people in the US have hypertension. The prevalence increases with age, and half of people over age sixty five have high blood pressure. 140/90 is generally considered to be the upper limits of normal, however 120-139/80-89 is considered to be prehypertension. Both the top number (systolic) and the bottom (diastolic) are important, but in people over age fifty, the systolic is more important as a risk factor for CHD. A diagnosis of hypertension should be made only after multiple readings are obtained. Having hypertension (and even prehypertension) increases the risk of heart failure, heart attack, stroke and kidney disease, whereas effective therapy reduces the risk of these complications.

For most patients, the goal of therapy will be readings under 140/90. For high risk patients, particularly those with diabetes or kidney disease, the guidelines recommend readings under 130/80. Some physicians are trying to get all their patients below 130/85. Many patients with hypertension are not at their BP goal.

For those with mild and uncomplicated hypertension, a trial of weight reduction, diet, and exercise should be done first, before considering medication. Reducing the intake of alcohol and salt is also beneficial. The best diet is the DASH diet which is described earlier in this book.

If medication is to be used, the guidelines suggest a thiazide diuretic as first line therapy, but some experts think that thiazides, by themselves, may not prevent strokes or heart attacks. After the initial steps, the doctor has a wide array of drugs to consider. Most patients need two or more drugs to achieve goal readings, and some drugs are combined in a single pill for convenience. Some antihypertensive drugs are specifically chosen because they have unique effects besides BP lowering that could help those with coexisting conditions such as heart failure.

Home blood pressure devices are an excellent idea for monitoring response to therapy, and I recommend a digital self-inflating machine such as by Omron® (www.omronhealthcare.com). If you are obese, get a "large" arm cuff. Omron machines come with a cuff that is suitable for arms that are 9"-17" in circumference. If needed, your doctor can arrange for a twenty four hour BP monitor to see how your BP varies over a full day. This test is very useful because of the wide fluctuations in readings that occur over 24 hours. It is a good technique to evaluate "white coat hypertension."

The best source of information on hypertension is the Seventh Report (2003) of the Joint National Committee (JNC 7) on Prevention, Detection, Evaluation and Treatment of High Blood Pressure (www. nhlbi.nih.gov). The Eighth Report is due out in late 2011.

Estrogen/Women's issues: Premenopausal women have a lower risk of CHD than men, but the risk becomes the same after the menopause. On the other hand, premenopausal women can be at increased risk for CHD if other risk factors such as smoking or diabetes are present. High triglycerides and low HDL levels seem to create a particularly high risk in women.

Although many older trials had suggested that hormone replacement therapy (HRT) with estrogens, after the menopause, would reduce the risk of coronary heart disease by one half, (*New England Journal* 325:756, 1991), recent data has dramatically changed the guidelines.

The Women's Health Initiative is a huge randomized trial which, in 2003, reported that the use of HRT increased the number of cardiovascular events. Subsequent results in the trial demonstrated that the issue is quite complex. Although doctors no longer prescribe HRT for most postmenopausal women, the use of estrogens seems to be protective in younger postmenopausal women and might still be used in selected patients. (HRT and the Young at Heart, *NEJM* 356:2639, June 21, 2007). This matter must be discussed with your physician.

The potential benefits of HRT in preventing heart disease in some patients are probably related to the effects on blood fats. The LDL cholesterol can be expected to drop 24% with HRT, while the HDL will rise an average of 7%.

The "Nurses Health Study" has evaluated **lifestyle practices** as they relate to cardiovascular risk in 84,129 women. The follow-up was for fourteen years, and they looked at heart attacks and coronary deaths over time. 41% of the cardiac events were attributable to smoking. Aside from not smoking, the lifestyle practices associated with the lowest risk were: diet with low consumption of transfats; high consumption of cereal fiber, fish oils and folic acid; a high dietary ratio of polyunsaturated to saturated fat; at least 30 minutes per day of moderate to vigorous exercise including brisk walking; a body mass index of under 25; and consumption of small amounts of alcohol (the equivalent of half a glass of wine). The investigators concluded that 82% of coronary events might have been prevented if all the women had fallen into the lowest risk group. (Stampfer *NEJM*, July 6, 2000).

The "Nurses Health Study" did not show a benefit from low fat diets, but the trial was not successful in convincingly drawing conclusions on this issue. It did suggest that for women, the type of fats consumed might be more important than the amount. A heart healthy diet is still the best choice for dietary prevention in both men and women.

Elderly: Clinical trials show that older patients benefit from lipid lowering therapy as much as younger patients do. (*Geriatrics*, May, 2000). The ATP guidelines say that two thirds of first major coronary events occur in persons over age 65, and many older people who have no cardiac symptoms are walking around with disease. In discussing prevention in this group, the guidelines recommend aggressive lipid therapy in older individuals who have multiple risk factors.

Younger patients: It is recommended that all adults over the age of 20 have their cholesterols checked once every 5 years. The idea is to identify young people at risk of atherosclerosis and to curtail its development early. Drug therapy is generally not recommended for men under age 35 and women under age 45. There is a trend now to begin medication for cholesterol in younger people who seem to be at high risk, however there is little data regarding risk of long term side effects. For young people at risk, life style changes should be tried first, but for someone at high risk, such as a strong family history of early CHD or a very high LDL cholesterol (e.g. over 190), then drug therapy will likely be needed sooner than later.

Diabetes is a major risk factor for cardiovascular disease. CHD occurs more frequently and at a younger age in diabetics. Diabetics often have high triglycerides and low HDL, and when combined with high LDL cholesterol, the risk becomes substantial. Diabetics often have other metabolic problems along with lipid abnormalities including insulin resistance, obesity, and increased blood clotting. Prevention of CHD in diabetics must be approached aggressively including control of lipids, weight, sugar and blood pressure.

Drug Therapy In Prevention: Focus On Cholesterol

*S*econdary prevention: Multiple research trials have verified that lowering blood cholesterol levels, particularly with statin drugs, in patients with preexisting coronary heart disease, will significantly reduce the risk of death, angina, heart attack, congestive heart failure, necessity for bypass surgery or angioplasty, and stroke. In addition, these studies show that the benefits can be documented within months of aggressive cholesterol lowering.

The most famous trial of this type was done in Scandinavia (The "4S Trial, *"Lancet,* 1994) in which cholesterol lowering with a statin drug called simvastatin (Zocor) resulted in a 42% reduction in risk of dying from CHD in over 4,000 patients with angina or prior heart attack. Other secondary prevention trials have found similar benefits in patients with preexisting CHD, and this even includes those who have cholesterol levels that are average for the American population. In the "LIPID Trial" (*NEJM*, 1998, 1349), over 6,000 men and women were studied, and benefits were found with the statin drug pravastatin (Pravachol) even with total cholesterols in the 155- 271 range.

The scientific data is so impressive, that some experts think that this therapeutic approach produces results as good as bypass surgery or angioplasty in terms of reducing risk of death and heart attack. The "AVERT" trial, done at the University of Michigan, showed that aggressive lowering of cholesterol, with medication, in patients with coronary disease, produced results at least as good as angioplasty in preventing events such as heart attack. (*NEJM*.1999; 341: 70).

Another drug trial of people who had prior bypass surgery found reduced graft closure when cholesterol was lowered aggressively with medication, and this benefit occurred regardless of age or gender. ("Post CABG Trial", *Circulation,*1999).

Despite such extraordinary research findings, it is estimated that large numbers of heart patients are being inadequately treated for their lipid problems, either by not being given statins at all, or by failing to achieve therapeutic goals.

Primary prevention: Similar benefits have been documented in apparently healthy individuals with high cholesterol. The most impressive study used medication to lower cholesterol levels. In the "West of Scotland Coronary Prevention Study" ("WOSCOPS", *NEJM*, 1995), over 6000 men, ages 45-64, with no history of CHD, but with high cholesterol, were studied. The treatment group received pravastatin (Pravachol) and had an over 30% reduction in risk of death from CHD and risk of heart attacks. The latest trials have even suggested an impressive benefit in certain healthy individuals who have normal blood cholesterol levels. A 2009 study of over 200,000 individuals in Israel (*Archives of Internal Medicine*) showed that healthy people who take statins have a major reduction in death rates. However, although the concept of using statin drugs to treat selected people who have no heart disease seems to be a reasonable approach, the idea remains a controversial and complicated issue.

Although lowering of LDL cholesterol levels has emerged as the most important goal in treating abnormal lipids, there is evidence that raising HDL levels will also be preventive, independently of LDL lowering. Studies show that the risk of CHD declines by 2-4% for every 1 mg. increase in HDL cholesterol (*Circulation*, 1989; 79:8). In a Veterans Administration trial of heart patients with normal LDL cholesterol, but low levels of HDL, treatment with a drug called gemfibrizole resulted in an elevation of HDL levels by 8% and a 22% reduction in risk of heart attacks and death. (*NEJM*,1999, 341:410). It is difficult to substantially raise blood HDL levels, and this subject is discussed later.

Goals of Therapy— How Low to Go: Researchers are not sure as to how low to take the cholesterol number. In recent years, the LDL goals have been reduced because of trials which suggest that "lower is better". The goal of therapy will vary depending on the risk profile of the patient and whether the issue is primary or secondary prevention. In high risk patients, aggressive therapy has been shown to reduce plaque in coronary and carotid arteries. In general, for healthy people (primary prevention) with no major risk factors, the total cholesterol goal should be 200-239 mg/dl, while the LDL should be 100-129 mg/dl. Individual goals will be different, and the highest risk patients need to be treated aggressively. Discuss your lab results with your doctor.

Physicians should follow the guidelines available from the National Cholesterol Education Program (NCEP Adult Treatment Panel III) regarding detection, evaluation and treatment of high blood cholesterol in adults, however, those guidelines are so complex and long (nearly two hundred pages), that it is unlikely that most doctors have read the entire document, and the practice of lipid management by doctors in the US is inconsistent and varies widely. In community practice, only one third of patients with hyperlipidemia are meeting standard treatment goals. The goals of ATP III were set in 2002, but were updated in 2004. Copies of the guidelines can be ordered or viewed online. (www.nhlbi.nih.gov)

Cholesterol lowering drugs: It is very difficult to achieve the cholesterol lowering goals recommended by the NCEP using diet and exercise alone. These goals can usually be met only with medications. The NCEP goals revolve around the LDL levels, which are considered the most important for prevention. Diet can usually lower cholesterol by about 5-15%, whereas cholesterol lowering drugs can lower it by 20-60% or more. In general, patients with heart disease should have LDL levels of under 100 mg/dl while those looking for primary prevention aim for 130 mg/dl. The most recent guidelines suggest LDL levels under 70 mg/dl in very high risk patients, such as those who already have known CHD. There is no evidence that lowering LDL to very low levels will cause harm.

At the *Framingham Cardiovascular Institute*, lowering LDL cholesterol to less than 80 mg/dl caused symptoms of angina or claudication to diminish. This kind of improvement can occur within 3 months of starting intensive cholesterol lowering therapy. (Castelli, *American Journal of Cardiology*,1998 Nov; 82:60T). In a trial from Canada, patients with acute coronary syndromes and high cholesterol were placed on statin therapy in the hospital. Treatment improved arterial function within 6 weeks of starting therapy. This is due to beneficial effects on the inner lining of the artery and is independent of benefits that occur over time in altering the fat laden plaques that clog arteries. (*Circulation*, 1999; June).

More recent trials have shown that very aggressive treatment with statin drugs, resulting in blood LDL cholesterol levels well under 80 mg/dl, could result in benefits including reduction in plaque progression. (*NEJM* 350:1562, April 8, 2004). A remarkable recent finding suggests that drug therapy might be warranted even in coronary patients with normal LDL cholesterol levels of 100 mg/dl or less.

Statin drugs (HMG-CoA reductase inhibitors) such as Zocor (simvastatin), Mevacor (lovastatin), Pravachol (pravastatin), Crestor (rosuvastatin), and Lipitor (atorvastatin) have been shown to produce major decreases in mortality, heart attack risk, and other cardiovascular end points by about 20-40%. The reduction in risk also includes a 20% reduction in stroke risk. (*NEJM*, 8/2000). There have been very large trials looking at over 30,000 patients that clearly document these benefits. In a review of 5 major trials, benefits were seen for women and for the elderly, in addition to the well documented benefits in men. (*JAMA*, 12/22/99).

Death rates are reduced by 21%, while risk of major coronary events is reduced by 31%, on average, with statin therapy in patients with CHD (secondary prevention) or those who are at risk for CHD (primary prevention). Statins achieve these benefits by lowering LDL cholesterol levels by 35%, but they also increase HDL levels by about 5%-10% and lower triglycerides as well. The benefits are seen not only in clinical endpoints such as mortality rates, but studies with electron beam CAT scanners have shown reduction in coronary plaque in patients treated with statins. (*NEJM*, 12/31/99). Similar benefits have been found in primary prevention (risk reduction when apparently healthy individuals are treated)

It is thought that statins "slow the progression and induce the regression of coronary atherosclerosis" (Maron, *Circulation*. Jan 18, 2000). They also have some actions that are poorly understood and are not related to their cholesterol lowering actions, such as prevention of spasm in diseased arteries.

Dr Antonio Gotto from Cornell Medical School said, "Statin drugs have had the greatest impact of anything I've seen over the past three decades" He added, "With wider application, they have the potential of making a tremendous dent in death and disability from coronary disease"

Do not fear the statins—they offer you a huge potential benefit in exchange for a low risk of side effects. Major side effects such as inflamed muscles and liver toxicity are extremely rare. There have been claims that statins may reduce cognitive function, but that concern has not been proven. The risk of side effects increases if multiple lipid drugs are used in combination. These risks should be discussed with your physician.

Ezetimibe (Zetia) is a drug that lowers LDL cholesterol levels by blocking fat absorption in the intestine. When ezetimibe is combined with simvastatin *(Vytorin)*, the LDL levels can be lowered further than with the statin alone, but the combination did not reduce the amount of arterial plaque any more than the statin alone. ("ENHANCE Trial" NEJM, April, 2008). Another trial looking at these two drugs is currently underway. Doctors often use ezetimibe when patients cannot tolerate statins. Note that there may be a cancer risk with this drug, and that is being studied.

Niacin (Vitamin B6) is a potent drug when used in large doses and it is the best agent for raising HDL levels by 15-35%; it also lowers LDL cholesterol and triglycerides. But when niacin is used in large doses, there is the potential for side effects, and a physician should supervise this therapy, even though you can buy large dose niacin over the counter. Slow release prescription preparations can offer reduced side effects and safety. Sometimes statins and niacin are used in combination for high risk patients, and a study showed regression of coronary narrowing with this dual therapy. In 2009, a small trial from Amsterdam showed that niacin was superior to Zetia in reducing plaque.

Fibrates for raising HDL: Gemfibrozil/Lopid or fenofibrate/Tricor can be beneficial in raising HDL and lowering triglycerides. A Veterans Administration trial ("VA-HIT": *NEJM*, 1999) looked at heart patients with normal cholesterol, low HDL and high triglycerides. The drug gemfibrizole raised HDL levels by 6% while producing a 34% reduction in serious coronary events. The treatment also reduced the risk of carotid artery disease and transient ischemic attacks/strokes. Fibrates have not been shown to reduce mortality. Fibrates can cause significant side effects, and many doctors are reluctant to prescribe them. They are considered to be "second line" therapy.

Combination therapy: Sometimes lipid modifying drugs are used in combination, because no one drug can normalize all the lipoproteins, (*CVR&R* Jan. 2000), but the combinations can increase the risk of side effects.

Aspirin: For individuals with known vascular disease, a small daily dose of aspirin (75-100 mg per day) can protect against heart attack and stroke. For primary prevention, low dose aspirin may be protective in some men. Women may not benefit from low dose aspirin for primary prevention, although a large trial of women did show a preventive effect after age 65. (*NEJM* March 31, 2005). The subject is debatable. Discuss your need for aspirin and the dose with your doctor.

Ace Inhibitors: This class of drugs has been used to treat high blood pressure and congestive heart failure, but research has shown that a particular ACE inhibitor (ramipril/Altace) can lower the risk of cardiac complications in patients with vascular disease. The "HOPE Trial" studied over 9,000 patients followed for nearly 5 years and found a 22% reduction in risk of heart attack, stroke or death from cardiovascular causes. (*NEJM.* January 2000). It appears that ACE inhibitors can influence the function of the blood vessel wall and thus may inhibit plaque formation and arterial spasm. These benefits are independent of the blood pressure lowering actions of these agents. Other studies have disputed this benefit (*NEJM* November 11, 2004), so if you have coronary disease or other vascular problems, ask your doctor about ACE inhibitors for prevention.

PART TWO:

Recipes

By Eileen Goldfinger, cook and food preparation educator

Introduction

*D*r. William Castelli, former medical director of the Framingham Heart Study, has pointed out that most American families prepare the same recipes over and over again. He notes that the American diet is too high in fats, and he encourages people to **learn new recipes** that are heart-healthy. If people are to stick to a heart-healthy diet, they must learn how to prepare meals that are both nutritious and tasty. In this section of "Prevention Does Work," you will find heart-healthy recipes that will surprise you with their nutritional quality, wonderful flavors, and ease of preparation.

The Pantry

The first step in the process of food preparation is to **set up a well stocked pantry** that provides you with the necessary ingredients to create delicious and healthy meals. Read the labels carefully when you are food shopping. Once you have set up your pantry, you can use the recipes in this book as a framework, and then adapt the recipes to your personal taste using the ingredients found in your food cupboard.

The pantry should contain a variety of vegetables, fruits, spices, condiments, grains, broths, pastas, heart healthy oils, vinegars, margarines, and low fat dairy products.

When fresh produce is not available, it is desirable to have a supply of canned and frozen fruits and vegetables. A wide assortment of canned **beans** add variety, color, and texture to many recipes. Beans are high in protein and fiber, while being low in fat.

Your meals will become more interesting when you stock unusual canned items such as artichokes, hearts of palm, papaya and mandarin orange pieces.

Essential ingredients include **fat free broth and stock,** because they offer a flavorful liquid for many recipes. I prefer Kitchen Basics® broths, both chicken and vegetable, because they, unlike many other low fat broths, are low in sodium. **Cooking wine** is another item that is useful, because it is available in many flavors and doesn't spoil quickly like drinking wine. **Spices** are used to enhance the flavor of food. Among the most popular are black pepper, cayenne pepper, garlic, chili powder, parsley, oregano, bay leaf, and paprika. **Vinegars**, in a variety of flavors, are especially useful in salad dressings. The best heart-healthy **oils** are extra virgin olive and canola. You can purchase these oils in spray form as a way to reduce calories.

I have sea salt and kosher salt in the pantry, but I rarely use it in my recipes. Many ingredients such as tomato sauce, cooking wine and stock already contain salt. Cooks should taste the food when done and make adjustments as needed. People can add their own salt at the table.

Tomatoes and tomato sauces in jars or cans add flavor, color and texture to many low fat recipes. Do not choose sauces that contain cheese or cream.

Pasta or rice may be used as the main ingredient for some recipes but are also used as side dishes. When preparing rice dishes, most people think of white rice, but there is a wide variety of interesting and flavorful rice to consider such as wild, basmati, saffron, or brown rice. **Grains** such as couscous, kasha, barley and polenta are good complements to main dishes.

Canned fish such as tuna, salmon, sardines, crab and clams are important staples in a pantry; however they should be packed in water or broth.

Dried vegetables such as mushrooms, peppers, tomatoes, and beans also add variety in the pantry.

I prefer fresh **meat, poultry and fish**, but it is convenient to have some on hand in the freezer. Some **soy** products can be substituted for ground meat, such as MorningStar Griller Crumbles® or Lightlife Smart Ground®. They are found in the refrigerated section of the grocery store.

Dairy products, use fat free or 2% milk, low fat or fat free cheeses, and egg substitutes such as Eggbeaters®. You should choose margarines that contain no trans-fats. Tub margarines that are made from heart healthy oils are preferable, particularly the ones that contain omega-3 fatty acids such as Smart Balance® Regular (with flax oil).

Chicken

Spanish Chicken

1 pound chicken breast, skinned, not boned, cut in quarters
6 chicken wings cut in half
4 chicken or turkey sausages, spicy (optional), quartered
4 tablespoons olive oil
1 large onion, diced
1 teaspoon paprika
1 28 ounce can of San Marzano plum tomatoes, crushed by hand
1 cup fat free chicken stock
3 tablespoons fresh parsley, chopped
1 10 oz. package of frozen green peas
¼ cup white wine
3 garlic cloves, minced
freshly ground pepper to taste
salt to taste

In a large deep frying pan, sauté sausage until brown on all sides. Remove sausage from pan and put aside. Drain and discard fat. Add olive oil to pan and heat. Season the chicken with black pepper and then brown in pan. After chicken has been browned on both sides, remove from pan and set aside. Add onions to the pan and sauté on low-medium heat until onions become translucent, approximately 5 minutes. Add garlic and cook for 2 more minutes. Return chicken and sausage to pan and then add chicken stock, wine, tomatoes and paprika. Cover the pan and cook at a simmer for one hour. Stir occasionally. Add the frozen peas and parsley and leave cover of pan ajar, cook for an additional 15 minutes. If you want this to be a spicy dish, add ½ teaspoon of cayenne pepper. Add salt and pepper.

Serve with saffron rice.

Serves 4

Chicken or Turkey Marsala

1 pound chicken or turkey fillets
1 cup fat free chicken broth
½ cup Marsala wine
2 tablespoons olive oil
1 pound fresh white mushrooms, sliced
3 cloves garlic, minced
1 small onion, minced
4 tablespoons fresh parsley, chopped
3 teaspoons corn starch
4 teaspoons water
freshly ground black pepper, to taste
salt to taste

Place fillets on a board, cover with plastic wrap or waxed paper, and pound with metal mallet to flatten. In a large, deep frying pan, heat oil. Brown fillets for 3 minutes on each side. Remove fillets and set aside. Add onion and garlic to pan. Sauté on a low-medium heat until the onion wilts. Add the wine and the broth to the pan a little bit at a time; stir and simmer. Mix the cornstarch and water together in a glass until the liquid is smooth. Add this liquid to the pan and continue to stir until the sauce is the consistency of maple syrup. Put the fillets back into the pan and add parsley and mushrooms. Cover the pan, leaving the top ajar, and continue to cook on low-medium heat until the mushrooms begin to soften. Add salt and pepper. Remove from heat and serve over wild rice.

Serves 4

Chicken Scarpiello

4 whole chicken breasts, skinned and quartered
3 bell peppers (red, yellow, orange), thinly sliced; discard seeds and ribs
1 pound white or cremini mushrooms, sliced
½ cup red wine
½ cup chicken broth
½ teaspoon ground black pepper
½ cup flour
¼ cup olive oil
12 small red potatoes, parboiled
2 28 ounce cans San Marzano whole plum tomatoes, quartered
2 onions, cubed
4 cloves garlic, minced
½ teaspoon garlic powder
1 cup tomato sauce (marinara or spicy)
freshly ground pepper to taste
salt to taste

Season flour with garlic powder and ½ teaspoon ground black pepper. Coat chicken quarters lightly in seasoned flour. Heat oil in a large frying pan or Dutch oven. Add chicken quarters and cook until pieces are browned on both sides. Remove chicken from pan. Add onions and bell peppers to the pan and sauté on medium heat until onion is translucent, 10 minutes. Add minced garlic and then cook for another two minutes. Place chicken pieces in pan with plum tomatoes, tomato sauce, red wine and broth, stir. Cover the pan, leaving the lid slightly askew, and simmer for 45 minutes. At this time add black pepper and salt to taste. Next, add the potatoes and the mushrooms. Simmer for an additional 15 minutes.

Serves 6

Eileen's Colorful and Spicy Chicken

1 pound chicken fillets, skinless, sliced into ½ inch pieces
½ red pepper, seeded and sliced
½ yellow pepper, seeded and sliced
1 large onion, halved and sliced
4 cloves garlic, minced
4 tablespoons olive oil
1 pound cremini or button mushrooms, sliced
1 cup chicken broth
½ cup white wine
¼ cup fresh parsley, chopped
6 leaves fresh basil, julienned
½ jalapeno pepper, thinly sliced, seeds and ribs removed
1 tablespoon cornstarch
3 tablespoons cold water
freshly ground black pepper to taste
salt to taste

In a large frying pan, heat olive oil on low-medium heat. Add chicken pieces and sauté on both sides for 2 minutes per side. Remove chicken from pan and set aside. Sauté onion and peppers for 10 minutes. Add garlic and cook for additional 2 minutes. Add wine, broth and black pepper. Stir and bring to a boil. After the sauce comes to a boil, reduce the heat to a simmer and cook for 7 minutes. In a glass, mix the cornstarch and the water; add to the pan and stir, causing the sauce to thicken. Now add the chicken fillets, mushrooms, parsley and basil to the sauce, cover pan and simmer for another 10 minutes.

Serve over rice.

Serves 4

"Feel Good" Chicken with Orange Sauce

Chicken:
2 chicken breasts, skinless and boneless
¼ cup orange liqueur (optional)
½ cup orange juice
1 tablespoons orange zest
2 tablespoons olive oil
2 tablespoons fresh thyme (remove leaves from woody stem)
freshly ground black pepper to taste
salt to taste

Sauce:
½ cup orange juice
2 tablespoons corn starch
¼ cup cold water
2 tbsp orange liquor (optional)

Preheat oven to 350 degrees.
Place chicken breasts on large wooden board and cover with clear wrap or waxed paper. Pound (the feel good part) with a flat metal mallet until flat. Combine all ingredients (listed under chicken section), including the chicken, in a large resealable bag. Marinate in the refrigerator for 1 hour. Then remove the breasts from the bag and place them in an oven proof dish. Place the marinade in a bowl. Bake chicken for 30 minutes, basting with marinade every 10 minutes.

While breasts bake, prepare the orange sauce: Put orange juice in a saucepan on low-medium heat, simmer. In a glass, mix corn starch with cold water and add it to the pan. Stir until orange juice thickens. Add the orange liquor now. Serve over chicken breasts.

Serves 2

Fish

Swordfish With Pasta

¾ pound swordfish steak, 1 inch cubes
1 jalapeno (hot) pepper, seeded and minced
1 small onion, diced
2 tomatoes, seeded and diced
4 tablespoons olive oil
2 cloves garlic, thinly sliced
1/3 cup white wine
½ pound pasta
1 teaspoon black pepper, freshly ground
3 tablespoons parsley, chopped
salt to taste

Heat olive oil in large frying pan on low-medium heat. Season swordfish cubes with ½ teaspoon black pepper and cook until brown on one side; turn over and brown other side. Remove fish from pan and set aside. Sauté pepper and onions for 10 minutes. Add garlic and cook for 2 minutes. Add tomatoes and wine; stir and simmer for 2 minutes. Return the fish to pan along with remaining black pepper, salt to taste, and parsley. Simmer in covered pan for 7 minutes.

While you are preparing the fish, cook the pasta according to the instructions on the box. When the pasta is done, drain it and place it in a large shallow bowl. Ladle the fish and sauce combination on top.

Serves 2

Shrimp Livornese

12 large shrimp, peeled and deveined
1 medium onion, diced
2 tablespoons olive oil
2 garlic cloves, thinly sliced
2 plum tomatoes, seeded and diced
10 black olives, pitted and sliced
¼ cup white wine
½ cup chicken broth
freshly ground black pepper to taste
salt to taste

Heat olive oil in a large frying pan on low-medium heat. Add shrimp and cook for 2 minutes on each side. Remove the shrimp from the pan and set aside. Sauté onion in the pan until soft. Add garlic and simmer for 2 minutes. Then add the remaining ingredients, except the shrimp, and sauté for 7 minutes with a cover on the pan. Add the shrimp and stir them into the sauce; cook for another 2 minutes.

Serves 2

Scallops and Shrimp Portuguese Style

1 pound sea scallops
16 large shrimp, peeled and deveined
4 tablespoons olive oil
1 tablespoon fresh lemon juice
¼ teaspoon cayenne pepper
¼ cup fresh parsley, chopped
¼ cup of white wine
3 tablespoons cognac or sherry
freshly ground black pepper to taste
salt to taste

In a large frying pan, heat oil on low-medium, add scallops and shrimp Cook for two minutes on each side. The scallops should brown on both sides and the shrimp should turn pink. With a slotted spoon, remove the seafood from the pan and set aside. Add garlic, lemon juice, cayenne pepper and white wine to the pan and sauté for 2 minutes. Add parsley, cognac, salt and pepper; stir and cook for 2 more minutes. Return the seafood to the pan together with any juices they released while set aside. Simmer seafood in sauce for 5 minutes. Serve over saffron or wild rice.

Serves 4

Stuffed Flounder

¾ pound flounder
¾ pound fresh, prewashed baby spinach
1 plum tomato, seeded and diced
1 shallot, diced
4 tablespoons olive oil
Olive oil spray
¼ teaspoon red pepper flakes
1 teaspoon ground garlic
2 tablespoons paprika
¼ cup white wine
freshly ground black pepper to taste
salt to taste

Preheat oven to 400 degrees.

Prepare stuffing:
Heat 2 tablespoons olive oil on low-medium heat in a frying pan; add spinach, and garlic; sauté until leaves begin to wilt. Remove spinach and garlic from the pan; place in a bowl. Add another 2 tablespoons olive oil to the pan and, on low-medium heat, add red pepper flakes, tomato and shallot. Sauté for 3 minutes. Remove the tomato mixture and add it to the bowl with the spinach. Add salt and pepper. Mix all ingredients together.

Prepare fish:
Evenly divide the stuffing and place it in the center of each fish filet. Bring the ends of fillet together around the filling and hold in place with a wooden toothpick. Sprinkle the stuffed fillets with paprika. Spray olive oil on the bottom of an ovenproof dish and add the white wine. Place the fish in the dish. Bake for 15 minutes.

Serves 2

Eileen's Spanish Cod Fish

¾ pound cod fillets
4 cloves of garlic, minced
1 medium onion, diced
½ jalapeno (hot) pepper, thinly sliced, seeds and ribs removed
¼ yellow pepper, cubed
¼ red pepper, cubed
6 San Marzano whole plum tomatoes, cubed
¼ teaspoon ground coriander
1/3 cup sherry
6 tablespoons olive oil
½ pound cremini or button mushrooms, sliced
freshly ground black pepper to taste
salt to taste

Preheat oven to 425 degrees.

Place 2 tablespoons olive oil in a fry pan on low-medium heat. Add onions and peppers. Sauté for 7 minutes. Add the garlic; sauté for an additional 2 minutes. Add tomatoes, coriander, sherry, salt and pepper; stir and cook for 10 minutes. Coat the bottom of a 9x11 baking dish with the remaining oil. Place cod fillets and mushrooms in the baking dish and pour sautéed vegetable sauce on top of the fish. Place dish on center rack in oven and bake at 425 degrees for 15 minutes or until the fish begins to flake.
Serve over rice.

Serves 2

Cod Fish with Orange Glaze and Mango Salsa

Fish:

Preheat oven 450 degrees

¾ pound cod fish (any meaty fish can be substituted for cod, such as salmon, swordfish or halibut)
¼ teaspoon freshly ground black pepper
¼ teaspoon chili powder
2 tablespoons olive oil

Heat oil in a nonstick frying pan on low-medium heat. Rub pepper and chili powder on both sides of fillets. Add the fish to the pan. Cook fillets until they are brown on one side; turn over and brown other side. Remove pan with fillets from stove and place in oven for 10 minutes.

Glaze:

½ cup orange juice
2 teaspoons corn starch
1/8 cup cold water

Place orange juice in a small saucepan and heat on a low-medium. In a glass, mix cornstarch and water until smooth; add to sauce pan. Stir until juice becomes thick.

Salsa:

2 mangoes, peeled and diced
½ jalapeno pepper, seeded and minced
1 roasted red pepper (available in jars, diced)
¼ teaspoon ground garlic powder
salt to taste
freshly ground black pepper to taste

Gently mix all salsa ingredients together. Serve fish over salsa and pour glaze on top of fish.

Serves 2

Sole Stuffed with Shrimp and Crabmeat

1 pound sole fillets (or flounder)
½ pound shrimp, deveined, peeled and cubed
10 ounces crabmeat
3 cloves garlic, minced
1 medium onion, minced
1 stalk celery, minced
½ cup white wine
1 teaspoon freshly ground black pepper
2 tablespoons fresh parsley, minced
½ a yellow bell pepper, julienne
½ red bell pepper, julienne
10 white mushrooms, thinly sliced
¼ teaspoon cayenne pepper
½ teaspoon paprika
6 tablespoons olive oil
½ cup of fish (or chicken) broth
1 teaspoon ground garlic
1 teaspoon lemon zest
2 tablespoon cornstarch
1/8 cup cold water

Fish:
Season both sides of the fillets with ground garlic, ½ teaspoon black pepper, and paprika. Set aside.

Preheat oven to 400 degrees.

Stuffing:
In a large fry pan, heat 2 tablespoons of olive oil on low-medium. Add onions and celery; sauté until they become translucent, approximately 5 minutes. Add half of the minced garlic, remainder of black pepper, cayenne pepper and ¼ cup of white wine. Stir and cook for another 7 minutes. Add crabmeat and shrimp and cook for 2 minutes, until shrimp turns pink. Remove from the heat.

Stuff the fillets:

Rub the remaining oil on a baking tray, place fillets on tray. Divide the stuffing equally in the center of each fillet. Roll the two ends of each fillet towards the center and hold in place with a wooden toothpick. Bake in oven for 15 minutes at 400 degrees.

While the fish is cooking, prepare the sauce.

Sauce:

In the pan used to make stuffing, add fish broth, and ¼ cup white wine, remainder of minced garlic, parsley, black pepper and lemon zest. Heat to a simmer and stir. In a glass, mix cornstarch and cold water until it is smooth and add to the pan. Cook and stir on a medium heat until the sauce begins to thicken. Add julienne peppers and mushrooms to sauce and simmer for 15 minutes. Serve over fish.

Serves 4

Grilled Salmon Steaks with Pepper Mayonnaise Sauce

2 1 inch thick salmon steaks (you can substitute two 6 ounce fillets)
¼ red bell pepper, julienned
¼ yellow pepper, julienned
2 scallions, sliced on an angle
½ green zucchini, julienned
4 tablespoons low fat mayonnaise
1 tablespoon fresh dill, minced
2 tablespoons low fat milk
1 clove garlic, minced
4 tablespoons olive oil
salt to taste
freshly ground black pepper to taste

Mix mayonnaise, dill, milk, garlic, salt and pepper in a bowl.
Remove a third of the sauce from the bowl and set remainder aside for later use.
Use a pastry brush and lightly brush the third of the sauce on both sides of the salmon
steaks.

Add 2 tablespoons of olive oil to a nonstick pan. Place fish in pan and cook on medium heat until the underside begins to brown; about 5 minutes. Flip the steak over and cook until the second side browns.

While the fish is browning, heat the remaining olive oil in a sauté pan; add peppers, scallions and zucchini. Sauté vegetables for 10 minutes on a low-medium heat. Add the remainder of the mayonnaise mixture to the vegetables; stir and cook for 5 minutes.

Serve the salmon fillets with the pepper mayonnaise sauce on top.

Serves 2

Salmon Croquettes

1 14 ½ ounce can of pink salmon (skinless and boneless)
2 ounces of Eggbeaters (or egg whites)
1 tablespoon fresh dill, minced
¼ cup seasoned bread crumbs
4 tablespoons of olive oil
¼ red peppers, julienned
¼ yellow pepper, julienned
1 fresh tomato, diced
1 small onion, minced
¼ teaspoon ground garlic
salt to taste
freshly ground black pepper to taste

Place the salmon in a bowl; chop until smooth. Add the Eggbeaters, salt, pepper, garlic, dill, and breadcrumbs to the salmon. Mix these ingredients together with your hands and form them into cakes. Heat 2 tablespoons of olive oil in a non-stick pan and add croquettes. Cook croquettes until one side browns; flip them over and brown on other side.

While the croquettes are cooking, heat remaining oil in another pan and sauté peppers, tomatoes and onions until they wilt; about 7 minutes. Serve with croquettes.

Serves 2

Salmon Fillets with Spicy Maple Syrup Sauce

¾ pound salmon fillets
4 tablespoons olive oil
½ teaspoon freshly ground black pepper
1 teaspoon ground garlic
2 tablespoons brown sugar
¼ cup maple syrup
¼ cup white wine (or broth)
¼ teaspoon of cayenne pepper

Preheat oven to 450 degrees.
Season salmon with ¼ teaspoon black pepper. Heat oil in a nonstick pan on medium heat. Cook fillets until underside browns; turn fish over and cook until other side is crispy.

While salmon is browning, place in a small sauce pan the remaining black pepper, garlic, brown sugar, cayenne pepper, maple syrup and wine; stir and bring to a boil.
Reduce heat and allow to simmer.

After the salmon has been browned, put 2 tablespoons of sauce on each fillet and put the pan with the fish in oven for 5 minutes.

Pour the remaining sauce on the fillets and serve.

Serves 2

Grilled Whole Red Snapper with Tomato Sauce

1 small whole red snapper
1 lemon cut in half (juice ½ the lemon and use in the sauce)
1 tablespoon low fat mayonnaise
1 tablespoon ground garlic
4 tablespoons olive oil
2 garlic cloves, minced
¼ cup white wine
¼ cup broth, vegetable or chicken
1/8 teaspoon red pepper flakes (more if you like spicy)
8 fresh basil leaves, julienned
2 plum tomatoes, seeded and diced
salt to taste
freshly ground black pepper to taste

Preheat grill on medium heat.

Fish:
Rinse the fish in cool water and pat dry. Rub ½ the lemon on both sides of the snapper; place lemon inside the fish. Sprinkle salt, pepper and ground garlic on both sides of the fish and in its cavity. Brush a thin coat of mayonnaise on both sides of the fish. This keeps the fish moist as it cooks.

Place fish in a barbeque basket designed for grilling fish. Grill the fish on medium to high heat for 10 minutes on each side or until the flesh begins to flake.

The fish can also be prepared in an oven. Preheat oven to 425 degrees. Prepare the fish as stated above and then place fish in a foil lined oven proof dish. Cook at 425 degrees for 10 minutes per side or until the flesh begins to flake. To crisp up the skin, place the fish under the broiler for 2 minutes.

Sauce:

Heat olive oil in a saucepan on low-medium heat and cook garlic for 2 minutes. Add the remaining ingredients, except the basil. Cook and stir sauce on a medium heat for 10 minutes.

Serve sauce over the grilled snapper and sprinkle with basil.

Serves 2

Shrimp with Penne Pasta and Spinach

1 small onion, diced
½ cup chicken broth
¼ teaspoon of ground garlic
1/8 teaspoon red pepper flakes
1 10 oz. package of fresh baby spinach, thoroughly washed
½ pound dry penne pasta
12 large shrimp, peeled and deveined
¼ cup white wine
4 tablespoons olive oil
salt to taste
freshly ground black pepper to taste

Cook pasta according to instructions on package, but undercook it by 3 minutes to make it al dente. Drain the pasta and put it aside.

Add oil to a large, deep fry pan and heat on a low-medium heat. Add onion; sauté for 5 minutes, then add the garlic, red pepper flakes, and ¼ cup chicken broth; cook for another 5 minutes. Add the shrimp to the pan; sauté for 2 minutes on each side. Remove the shrimp from the pan, but leave the onion and broth in the pan.

Add the spinach, white wine, remainder of broth, salt and pepper to the pan. When the spinach begins to wilt, add the pasta and the shrimp; toss and heat on medium heat for 5 minutes.

Serves 2

Vegetarian Dishes

Eggplant Parmesan

1 medium eggplant, peeled and very thinly sliced
¾ cup Eggbeaters ®
1 cup seasoned breadcrumbs
1 26 ounce jar marinara sauce
1 16 ounce package of fat free mozzarella cheese, sliced in ¼ inch pieces
¼ cup Parmesan cheese, grated

Preheat oven to 325 degrees.

Place Eggbeaters® and breadcrumbs in individual bowls.
Coat the bottom of a 9x11 oven proof casserole dish with a thin layer of tomato sauce.
Dip one slice of eggplant in Eggbeaters®, allowing excess to drip off before placing eggplant slice in breadcrumbs. Cover both sides of eggplant with breadcrumbs and place on the bottom of the casserole dish. Repeat this step until the casserole dish has a single layer of coated eggplant on the bottom. Next put a thin coat of tomato sauce on this layer. Cover the sauce with slices of mozzarella in a single layer and sprinkle this with some of the Parmesan cheese.

Repeat this process (each layer has eggplant, sauce and cheese) until you have used all the eggplant. Save enough mozzarella to cover the top of the casserole.
Cover the casserole dish with foil. Add several slits in the foil to allow steam to escape as the eggplant cooks.
Place casserole in the 325 degree oven; bake until the cheese melts and the eggplant becomes soft. This will take about 1 ½ hours.
Remove the foil; raise the oven temperature to 425 degrees and cook for another 15 minutes.

Serves 4

Twice Baked Potato

2 Idaho (russet) potatoes
2 tablespoons olive oil
½ teaspoon ground garlic
4 tablespoons Smart Balance® margarine
2 ounces low fat milk
2 ounces low fat mozzarella cheese (optional)
1 tablespoon paprika
salt to taste
freshly ground black pepper to taste

Preheat the oven to 450 degrees. Wash and dry potatoes, make two small slits on each side. Rub potatoes with oil and sprinkle with garlic. Place in the oven for 60 minutes. The potato is done when a knife can penetrate easily.

Remove the potatoes from the oven and cut a slit in each one lengthwise. Scoop the insides of the potatoes out with a spoon, making sure you do not tear the skins. Place the flesh of the potatoes in a bowl and, using a potato masher, make the potatoes as smooth as possible. Add margarine, salt, pepper and low fat milk. At this time you can also add some shredded low fat cheese to the mix. Divide the mix in half; put it into skins. Sprinkle top of each potato with paprika.

Lower the oven to 350 degrees. Place potatoes on a tray and put them back in the oven to reheat. Heat for 15 minutes.

Serves 2

Vegetarian Sloppy Joes

4 tablespoons olive oil
4 vegetarian burgers (found in the frozen food section of your market)
1 medium onion, diced
1 fresh tomato, cubed and seeded
½ teaspoon garlic powder
¼ cup white wine
¼ cup vegetable broth
1 small package fresh mushrooms, sliced
¼ cup tomato sauce
salt to taste
freshly ground black pepper to taste
½ cup low fat mozzarella cheese, shredded
2 large sub rolls or 4 small rolls

Cook the burgers according to the directions on the box. Using a hand chopper; chop burgers so that they resemble ground meat. Heat oil in a nonstick fry pan on low-medium. Add the onion, garlic and tomato; sauté for 5 minutes. Add the remaining ingredients (including the chopped burgers), except the mozzarella and rolls; increase the heat to medium; stir and cook for 10 minutes. Add the mozzarella; cook for another 5 minutes or until the cheese begins to melt. Place the mixture in the rolls and enjoy.

Serves 2

Ratatouille

1 eggplant, medium size, peeled and cubed
1 28 ounce can of whole plum San Marzano tomatoes, drained
½ yellow pepper, seeded and cubed
½ red pepper, seeded and cubed
1 onion, medium size, cubed
1 shallot, minced
2 cloves garlic, thinly sliced
½ cup of vegetable broth
¼ cup white wine
8 tablespoons olive oil
1 teaspoon dried oregano
10 fresh basil leaves, julienned
1 pound white or baby portabella mushrooms, quartered
salt to taste
freshly ground black pepper to taste

Place eggplant pieces on a lined baking tray; toss with 4 tablespoons olive oil. Bake in a 350-degree oven, until the eggplant is fork tender; approximately 15 minutes.

In a large, deep fry pan, add remaining olive oil; heat on low-medium. Add onion, garlic and shallot. Sauté until onion becomes translucent; approximately 5 minutes. Add all the remaining ingredients, except the liquids and eggplant, then sauté for 15 minutes or until vegetables have softened. Add the eggplant and liquids; stir and season with salt and pepper to taste. Raise the heat to medium. Cook for 10 minutes.

Serve over couscous, rice, noodles or pasta.

Serves 2

Cole Slaw

½ head green cabbage, shredded
1 medium carrot, shredded
1 small onion, diced
½ bell pepper (any color), diced
½ teaspoon ground garlic
¼ cup low fat mayonnaise
5 tablespoons white or cider vinegar
salt to taste
freshly ground black pepper to taste

Mix all the ingredients together in a large bowl. Cover and put in the refrigerator for an hour. Taste to adjust seasoning and serve.

Serves 4 to 6

Cholesterol Free Egg Salad

4 large eggs, hard boiled
2 tablespoons white vinegar
½ cup Eggbeaters®
1 tablespoon Smart Balance® margarine
1 stalk of celery, diced
2 tablespoons low fat mayonnaise
salt to taste
freshly ground pepper to taste

Place eggs in a sauce pan; cover with cold water; add vinegar. Cover pot and bring water to a boil. When the water has boiled, turn off the heat and keep the eggs in covered pot with the hot water for 15 minutes. Remove the eggs from the water and submerge them in ice water until they are no longer hot; then peel them. Separate the egg whites and discard the yolks. Set aside the whites.

Place margarine in a non stick pan on low-medium heat. Add the Eggbeaters® and cover the bottom of pan to create an omelet. Cook on both sides until omelet is well done. Allow the omelet to cool; cut into small pieces.

Place the whites of the hard boiled eggs into a bowl and chop into small pieces. Add the omelet pieces and the other ingredients into the bowl. Mix; taste and adjust seasoning.

Serves 2

Boboli® Vegetarian Pizza

1 10 inch Boboli® thin crust pizza or 2 Indian naan breads
1 8 ounce package low fat mozzarella cheese, sliced
1 cup marinara tomato sauce
¼ jalapeno pepper, thinly sliced, seeds removed
4 artichokes hearts, quartered (canned)
4 asparagus, peeled and cut on the diagonal in ½ inch pieces
½ teaspoon garlic powder
¼ teaspoon red pepper flakes
½ teaspoon dry oregano
freshly ground black pepper to taste
6 cremini mushrooms, thinly sliced
2 tablespoons extra olive oil
¼ cup Parmigiano Reggiano cheese (grated)

Heat the oven to 450 degrees.
Line the lower rack with tin foil to protect oven from drips.
Place a second rack in the middle of the oven.

Spread the tomato sauce on the Boboli® crust (or naan bread) with the back of a spoon so that it covers the entire crust. Layer the mozzarella cheese on top of the sauce. Arrange the vegetables on the cheese (you can substitute any low fat toppings that you like such as soy pepperoni, onions, bell peppers, and broccoli, tuna or anchovies). Sprinkle the seasonings on the vegetables. Sprinkle grated Parmigiano on top. Drizzle olive oil on top.
Place the pizza directly on the upper oven rack.
Cook for 10 minutes.

Serves 2

Serve with a mixed green salad.

Eggplant Casserole

1 small to medium sized purple eggplant, peeled and very thinly sliced
1 cup tomato sauce
6 cremini mushrooms, thinly sliced
8 asparagus; snap off bottoms
8 ounces fat free or low fat mozzarella cheese
4 ounces nonfat ricotta
4 tablespoons olive oil
½ cup seasoned breadcrumbs
1 tablespoon ground garlic
½ teaspoon red pepper flakes (to taste)
freshly ground black pepper to taste
1 tablespoon dry oregano

Preheat oven to 325 degrees.
Coat bottom of an oven proof casserole dish with olive oil. Layer the bottom of the dish with a single layer of eggplant slices. Cover the slices with half the tomato sauce, mozzarella cheese, ricotta cheese, seasoning and breadcrumbs. Repeat this step, making a second layer. Top this layer with mushrooms and asparagus.
Cover the dish with tin foil; make several slits in the tin foil to allow the steam to escape.
Bake in the oven at 325 degrees for 1 hour until the eggplant is fork tender and the mozzarella has melted.

Serves 2

Serve with a mixed salad and Italian bread.

Soups

Jewish Chicken Soup

1 4 pound whole chicken, quartered, skinned
1 large onion, diced
3 stalks celery, diced
4 carrots, peeled
2 cubes chicken bouillon
1 bunch fresh dill
1 bunch fresh flat-leafed parsley
4 tablespoons vegetable oil
water
½ teaspoon freshly ground black pepper to taste
salt to taste

Heat oil in an 8 quart stock pot; add onions and celery; sauté for 10 minutes, until they wilt. Cut 2 carrots into rounds and 2 carrots lengthwise and then in half. Add carrots to pot. Add chicken to pot and fill with water two inches above the chicken.
Bring to boil and then reduce heat to a simmer. Take ½ of the dill and parsley, tie them together with cotton twine and place in pot. Break bouillon cubes into pieces and add to pot. Add ½ teaspoon black pepper to pot; stir. Place cover on pot, leaving it ajar; simmer for 1 hour.
Remove dill and parsley from soup and discard. Remove the lengths of carrot from pot, mash them and put them back into pot.
Taste soup; add more pepper and salt according to taste. Add 4 tablespoons of chopped dill to soup.

Serve with cooked thin noodles or matzo balls. (Matzo balls can be purchased in the kosher, refrigerated section of some grocery stores).

Options:

Remove the chicken pieces after the soup has cooked; shred and debone the chicken and put the shredded pieces into the soup.

Add any vegetables and/or beans to the soup while it is cooking for another version of chicken soup.

Serves 4

Italian Fish Soup

1 28 ounce can San Marzano whole plum tomatoes, crushed by hand
6 small red potatoes, parboiled
4 cloves garlic, minced
1 medium onion, minced
1 small jalapeno pepper, seeded and minced
2 tablespoons freshly squeezed lemon juice
6 tablespoons olive oil
1 shallot, diced
3 cups broth (vegetable, chicken or fish)
1 cup hot water
½ cup white wine
½ head escarole, wash and separate leaves
1 can cannelloni beans, drained
10 large shrimp, peeled and deveined
½ pound fish: 1 inch cubes of any solid fish such as salmon, swordfish or halibut, or any combination of fish
salt to taste
freshly ground black pepper to taste

Heat 3 tablespoons of oil in 5 quart stock pot. Sauté onion, pepper, shallots and garlic for 2 minutes or until they begin to soften. Add tomatoes and continue to simmer for 10 minutes. Add the liquid and the remaining ingredients, except the fish, potatoes and escarole. Stir and simmer for 20 minutes.

While the soup is cooking, heat remaining oil on low-medium in a fry pan. Add the fish and shrimp; sauté for 2 minutes on each side.

Add shrimp, fish, potatoes and escarole to soup in stock pot. Stir and simmer for 15 minutes.

Taste to adjust seasoning.

Serve with a green salad and a baguette.

Serves 4

Spicy Shrimp and Escarole Soup

2 medium onions, diced
3 cloves of garlic, minced
¼ teaspoon red pepper flakes
1 head of escarole, coarsely chopped (discard outside leaves, wash remainder very well)
12 large shrimp, peeled and deveined
3 cups of chicken broth
½ cup fresh parsley, chopped
½ cup white wine
1/8 cup water
2 cans cannellini beans, drained (save liquid)
4 tablespoons olive oil
salt to taste
freshly ground black pepper to taste

In a small, non-stick pan, heat 2 tablespoons olive oil on low-medium. Add shrimp and a third of the minced garlic; cook shrimp for 2 minutes on each side. Place the garlic and shrimp on a plate and set aside. Leave the empty pan for a subsequent step.

In a 4-5 quart stockpot, add remaining olive oil and onion; sauté on low-medium heat until the onion becomes translucent. Add the remainder of the minced garlic and sauté until the garlic begins to soften (do not brown because the garlic will become bitter). Add one can of the cannellini beans that have been partially mashed with a fork, ¼ cup of parsley, and the red pepper flakes. Slowly add the liquid ingredients and stir. Turn the heat up to medium, so that the soup begins to simmer.

As the soup is simmering, reheat the pan that was used for the shrimp. Add 1/8 cup of water, turn the heat to medium, add the washed escarole, and cook until the escarole begins to wilt.

Add to the stock pot the remaining can of cannelloni beans, including the bean liquid; cooked shrimp; escarole; salt and pepper. Simmer for 10 minutes. Garnish with parsley.

Serve with a green salad and an Italian or French bread.

Serves 4

Seafood Chowder with Red Potatoes

6 tablespoons olive oil
1 tablespoon Smart Balance© margarine
2 tablespoons fresh parsley, minced
1 medium onion, diced
8 small red potatoes, parboiled and quartered
3 garlic cloves, thinly sliced
½ ancho pepper, seeded, thinly sliced
9 San Marzano canned whole plum tomatoes, diced
2 medium carrots, peeled and diced
1 celery stalk, thinly sliced
6 large scallops cut in half
12 large shrimp, peeled and deveined
2 6 ½ ounce cans minced clams, drained
2 cups chicken broth
1 cup clam broth
½ cup water
freshly ground black pepper to taste
salt to taste

In a 5 quart stock pot, heat 3 tablespoons of olive oil on medium heat; add onion, carrots and celery until they begin to soften, approximately 10 minutes. Lower the heat to low-medium, add garlic and ancho pepper, and sauté for 2 minutes. Add the tomatoes; stir and cook for 10 minutes. Raise the heat to medium. Add chicken broth, clam broth and water slowly; stir while you do this. Simmer liquid for 45 minutes; stir occasionally.

While the soup is simmering, add remaining olive oil and margarine to a non-stick pan; heat on low-medium. Add shrimp and scallops; cook for 2 minutes on each side. Set them aside.

After the soup has been cooking for 45 minutes, taste the broth to adjust seasoning.

Add black pepper and salt, if necessary. Add clams, shrimp, scallops and potatoes to the broth; simmer for another 10 minutes. Add parsley.

Serve with a green salad and French or Italian bread.

Serves 4

Turkey

Turkey Meatballs and Cannellini Beans

Meatballs:
2 tablespoons olive oil
1 pound ground white meat turkey
2 tablespoons garlic powder
½ teaspoon cayenne pepper
½ cup Eggbeaters
½ cup seasoned bread crumbs
¼ cup water

Sauce:
1 15 ounce can cannellini beans
½ cup chicken broth
2 tablespoons of ketchup
1 tablespoon ground garlic
¼ teaspoon freshly ground black pepper (to taste)
2 fresh tomatoes, seeded and diced

Preheat oven to 350 degrees.

Mix meatball ingredients together, except the oil. Wet your hands so the meat will not stick to them; form golf ball sized meatballs. Heat oil on low-medium, in a large frying pan. Add meatballs to the pan and brown on all sides. Remove meatballs from the pan; set pan aside for later use. Place meatballs in a single layer in an oven proof dish.
Bake in oven at 350 degrees for 15 minutes.

While the meatballs are baking in the oven, reheat the pan in which you browned the meatballs. Add chicken broth and half of the liquid from the can of beans into the pan, combining the liquid with the browned pieces of turkey that were left in the pan. Add garlic, black pepper and ketchup; then stir. Cook on low-medium heat for 2 minutes. Add diced tomatoes and stir. Simmer for 7 minutes until tomatoes start to soften. Add all the beans and remainder of liquid from the can. Cook and stir mixture for 5 minutes. Add meatballs to the pan and simmer for 5 minutes.

Serves 2-4

Healthy Meatballs-Italian Style

4 tablespoons olive oil
1 pound ground white meat turkey
2 tablespoons garlic powder
¼ cup Eggbeaters®
¼ cup dried parsley
1 tablespoon dried oregano
¼ teaspoon red pepper flakes
1 cup white bread, no crust, 1 inch pieces
¼ cup water
½ teaspoon freshly ground black pepper
salt to taste

In a large bowl, mix all the above ingredients together, except the oil, until they are all blended. Wet your hands so the meat does not stick to them; form golf ball sized meatballs. Brush olive oil on an ovenproof tray and place meatballs on the tray. Bake in oven at 350 degrees for 30 minutes, turning the meatballs once, so they cook on both sides. Check the inside of the meatballs to determine if they are fully cooked.

Serve with tomato sauce and pasta.

Serves 2-4

Chili (with or without meat)

1 28 ounce can of San Marzano whole plum tomatoes, drained and diced
1 cup of tomato sauce
4 tablespoons olive oil
1 medium onion, diced
1 red bell pepper, diced and seeded
1 yellow bell pepper, diced and seeded
2 cloves garlic, peeled and minced
3 15 ounce cans of beans; a variety gives an interesting look and texture to the dish (such as cannellini, red kidney, pink beans or black beans), drain
½ cup red wine
½ cup chicken or vegetable stock
½ teaspoon dry oregano
2 tablespoons fresh parsley, minced
¼ teaspoon red pepper flakes (to taste)
1 pound of ground turkey or chicken
(Instead of meat, you can use one of the soy products listed in the pantry section of this book.)
½ teaspoon of freshly ground black pepper
salt to taste

Heat oil in a large, heavy frying pan that is two or three inches deep and has a cover. If you are using meat or soy, add it to the pan now. Cook on low-medium heat until meat is brown. Remove meat from pan and set it aside.

The following steps are for the recipe, regardless if you use meat or not:

In the same pan, sauté onion, garlic and peppers until they wilt. Add tomatoes and tomato sauce; stir and cook on simmer for 15 minutes. Stir in wine, stock, spices; cook for 10 minutes. Add the beans and meat (or soy). Cover the pan, leaving the cover slightly ajar and simmer for 1 hour. If the chili is too thick add more broth.

Serves 2

Options:
You can add other vegetables to the chili for additional color and flavor such as frozen peas, canned or fresh corn or squash.

Sauce

Eileen's Hot and Spicy Tomato Sauce

4 tablespoons olive oil
1 26 oz jar of marinara tomato sauce
1 28 oz can of San Marzano whole plum tomatoes, crushed by hand
3 cloves of garlic, thinly sliced
1 medium onion, diced
½ teaspoon red pepper flakes (adjust to taste)
½ cup chicken broth
¼ cup red wine
2 teaspoons dry oregano
2 tablespoons fresh parsley, minced
8 leaves fresh basil, julienned
½ teaspoon freshly ground black pepper
salt to taste

Heat olive oil in a 5 quart Dutch oven on low-medium heat; add onion. Cook until onion wilts, about 10 minutes. Add garlic; cook for another 2 minutes. Add tomato sauce and plum tomatoes to the pot. Stir and simmer for 10 minutes. Add the rest of the ingredients, except the parsley and basil. Stir and simmer for 20 minutes. Taste to adjust seasoning. Add parsley and basil; cook for another 10 minutes.

Meat sauce:
Use 1 pound of ground turkey or chicken. Instead of meat, use Lightlife Smart Ground® or MorningStar Grillers Crumbles®. Both are soy based products and look like ground cooked meat. Brown the meat as the first step in the above recipe. Then proceed by adding the onion (see above).

Serves 4

Salad Dressing (vinaigrette)

¼ cup olive oil
4 tablespoons champagne vinegar or freshly squeezed lemon juice
¼ teaspoon garlic powder
1/8 teaspoon salt
¼ teaspoon freshly ground black pepper

In a small bowl, add salt, pepper, garlic powder and vinegar or lemon juice, stir.
Slowly drizzle olive oil into mixture and whisk together. Taste to adjust flavor.

Variations:
Add ¼ teaspoon of creamy Dijon mustard to the dressing.
Add 5 tablespoons of freshly grated Parmigiano Reggiano cheese to the dressing.
Add 1 teaspoon of low sodium soy sauce to the dressing.
Add ½ teaspoon of anchovy paste to the dressing (this plus Parmigiano Reggiano cheese will taste like a Caesar dressing).

Enough for two small salads.

Index

References

Dr. Dean Ornish's books such as "Reversing Heart Disease", "Eat More, Weigh Less", or "Everyday Cooking"_are excellent for understanding how to successfully initiate a strict low fat eating style. His books contain excellent recipes that illustrate how low fat cooking can be delicious. Try his soups or vegetable stew.

Dr. David Kessler, "The End of Overeating: Taking Control of the Insatiable American Appetite" (Rodale, 2009)

The **"Nutrition Action Health Letter"** put out by the Center for Science in the Public Interest: CSPI (PO Box 96611, Washington DC 20009- this newsletter has over one million subscribers.

"Harvard Men's Health Watch" newsletter (PO Box 420097, Palm Coast, Florida 32142-8894) and **"Harvard Women's Health Watch"** PO Box 420235 Palm Coast Florida 32142-0235

National Cholesterol Education Program (NCEP)—Third report of the Expert Panel on Detection, Evaluation, and Treatment of High Blood Cholesterol in Adults; ATP III—Adult Treatment Panel III. 2002 (National Heart, Lung and Blood Institute, National Institutes of Health) Contact them for a copy of this report. The ATP reports are available on the NHLBI website (www.nhlbi.nih.gov)

"Preventive Cardiology" by Joann Foody, MD

American Heart Association: http://www.americanheart.org
   Food and Drug Administration: http://www.FDA.gov/cder

Medical Journals:
   New England Journal of Medicine (NEJM)
   Journal of the American Medical Association (JAMA)
   Journal of the American College of Cardiology (JACC)

Circulation (published by the American Heart Association)
American Journal of Cardiology.(AJC)

Recipes: Try some of the attached recipes in Part 2 of this book. They are all low in fat, and Eileen Goldfinger has prepared all of them in our home, and I have enjoyed all of them. Learn to cook properly and you won't feel deprived.